COCONUT

OIL HEALTH BENEFITS

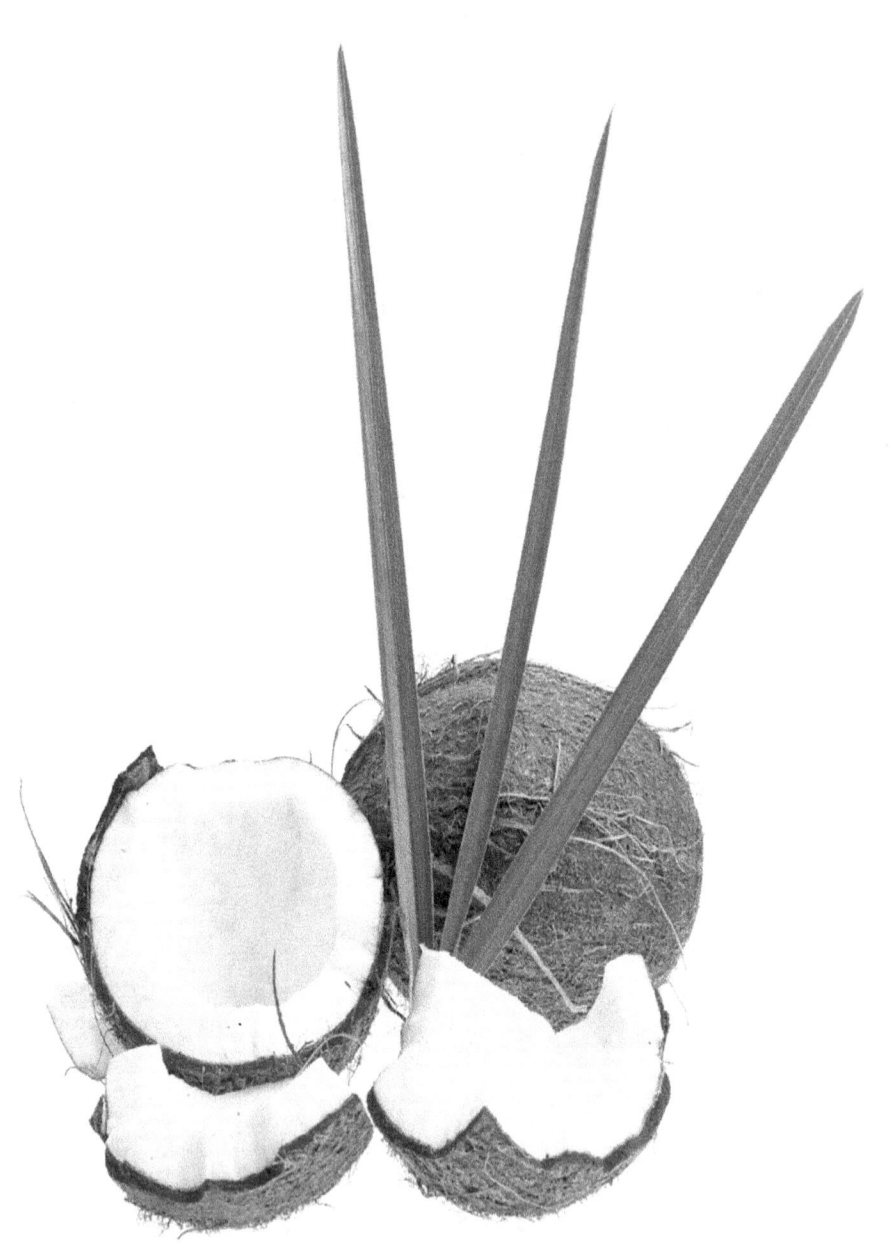

COCONUT OIL HEALTH BENEFITS

NICOLE K FREEMAN

First Printing, 2015

ISBN-13: 978-1514776674

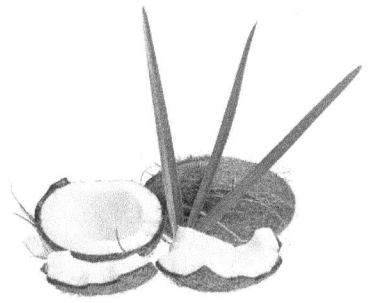

Contents

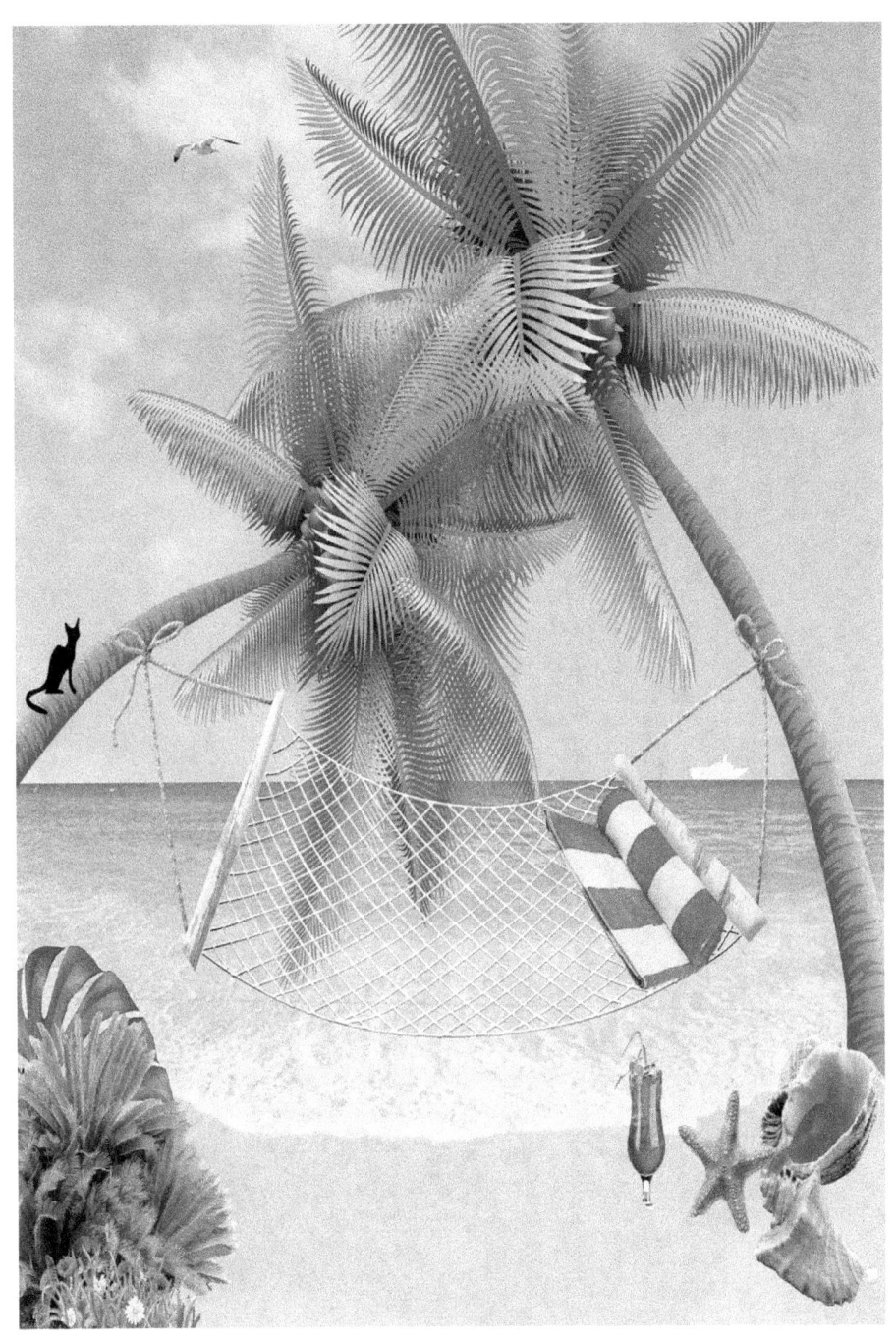

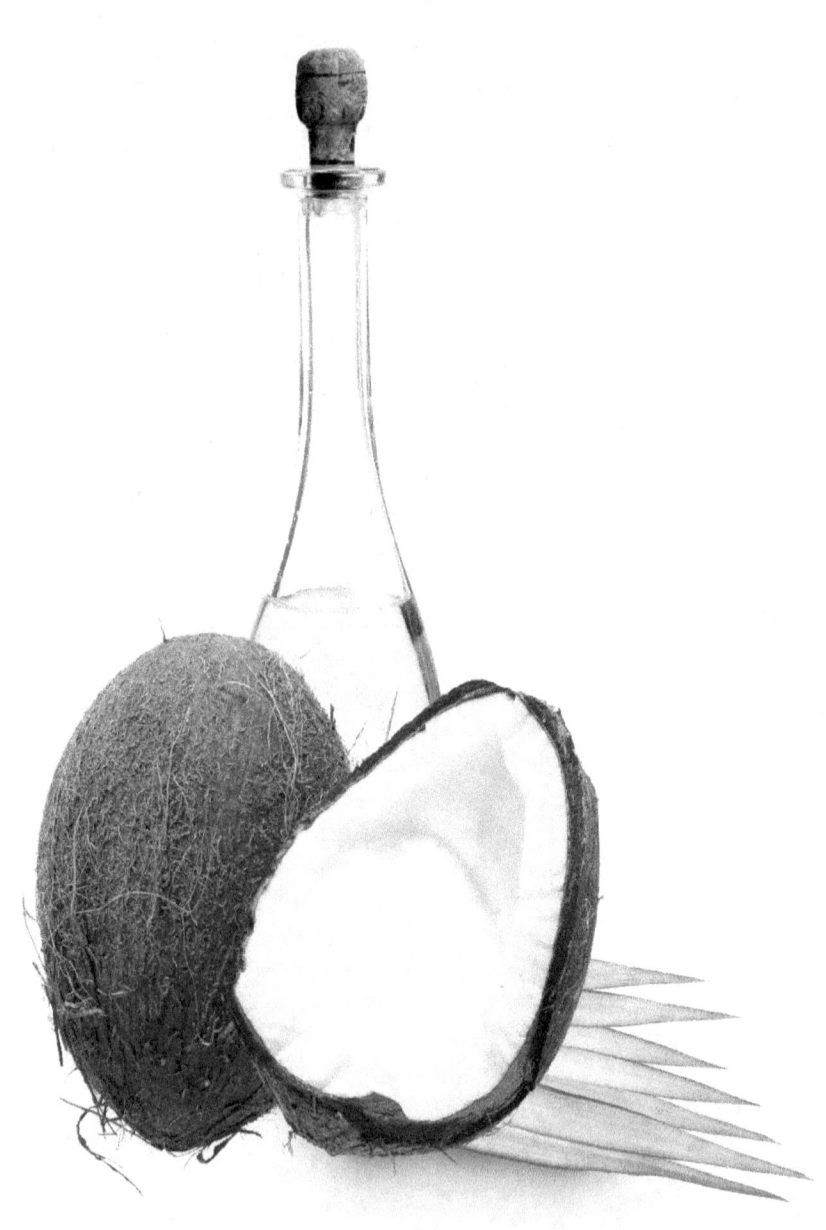

COCONUT OIL HEALTH BENEFITS

LOSE WEIGHT - BOOST ENERGY - PREVENT HEART DISEASE - BEAUTIFY SKIN AND HAIR

With Over 30 Recipes

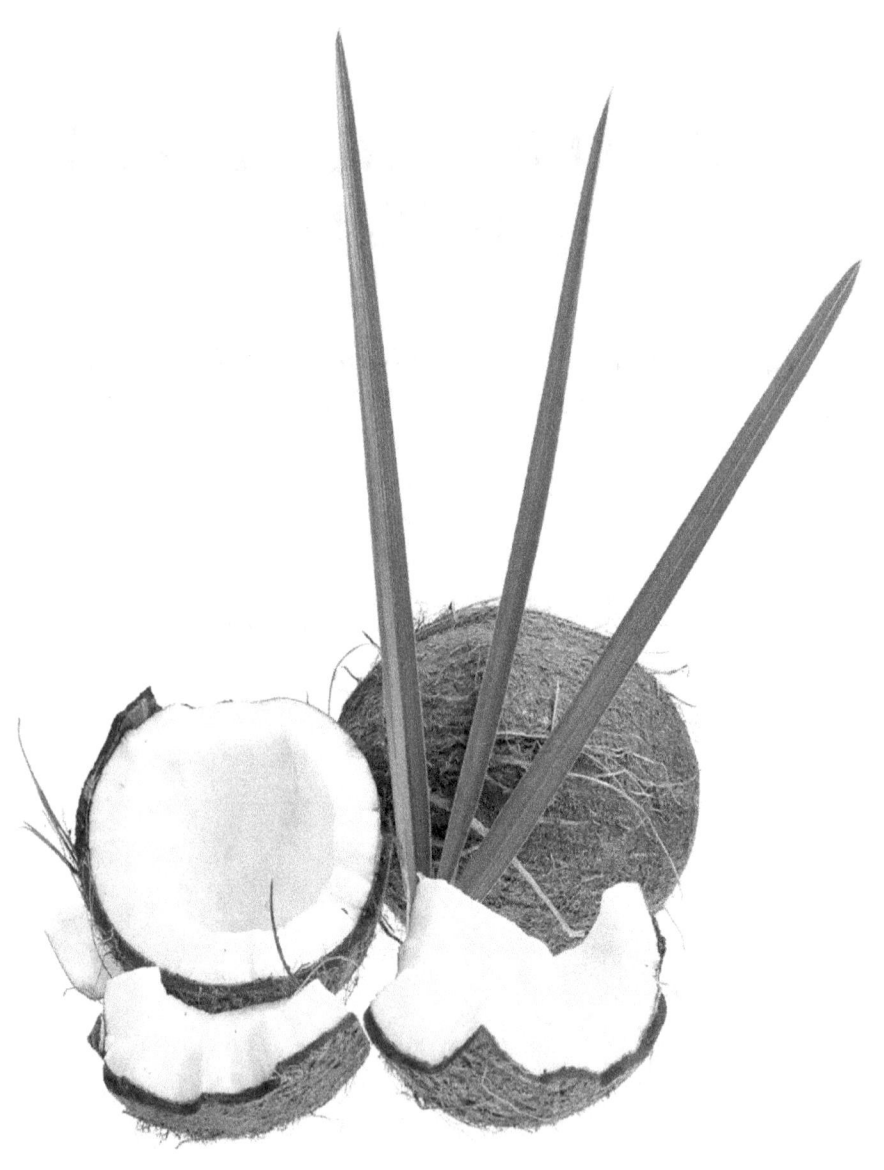

INTRODUCTION

In the past 4000 years of documented history, only one fruit has been used as an effective pharmaceutical and food. It has been nearly 3960 years that the coconut palm fruit has been used effectively at healing and nourishing people. Today, the oil is even used in some industrial applications.

Coconut oil has long been used around the world. From India to Africa and from South and Central America to Asia and Polynesia, the uses of the oil are widely documented. In Ayurvedic medicine, Sanskrit transcripts from 1500 BC document the oil as helping the body, mind and the soul.

Even explorers from Europe noted the effective use of the oil by people in the Pacific region. It was used every day for beauty and for nourishment. In World War Two, water from the young green coconut was used as a substitute for a saline drip. This saved the lives of many soldiers.

After World War Two, the oil was sold in England as margarine. In the United States, it was sold as coconut butter. It was not until the early 1950s, that it was cautioned against being consumed. A doctor alerted the public to the fact that fats in foods, especially saturated ones, were connected to heart disease. That ended using coconut oil for cooking temporarily.

It took decades for coconut oil to overcome its bad reputation. This is because it took time for there to be an awareness of the different types of saturated fats. Not all saturated fats it turns out are bad for human health. There are now three different categories of saturated fats and among the healthier fats is coconut oil.

Coconut oil has been shown in recent research that it is unique in its makeup. It has a medium chain of fatty acids that closely resembles that found in human breast milk. This is one reason coconut oil is found in baby formulas as well as sports drinks and even energy bars.

It is often listed as a medium chain triglyceride or MCT on product labels. This type of listing actually hides the fact that a form of the oil is being used in various products. It is important to note that medium chain fatty acids are easy for the human body to digest than those found in other oils.

It has been found that other oils like vegetable oils are easily damaged by heat. This makes them unhealthy to cook with as it causes them release free radicals that contribute to nearly 60 health complaints.

Coconut oil has been found to be easier to cook with and to digest. It is easy on the digestive system and, because it is easy to digest, it is also helpful in getting other nutrients to absorb into the body. One reason this fact was not discovered until recently is that most tests were done on hydrogenated coconut oil.

This type of oil does contain dangerous Trans Fats. Virgin pressed coconut oil is stable and resists the generation of free radicals when heated at high temperatures. This makes it extremely safe to use for cooking.

A UNIQUE TYPE OF FAT

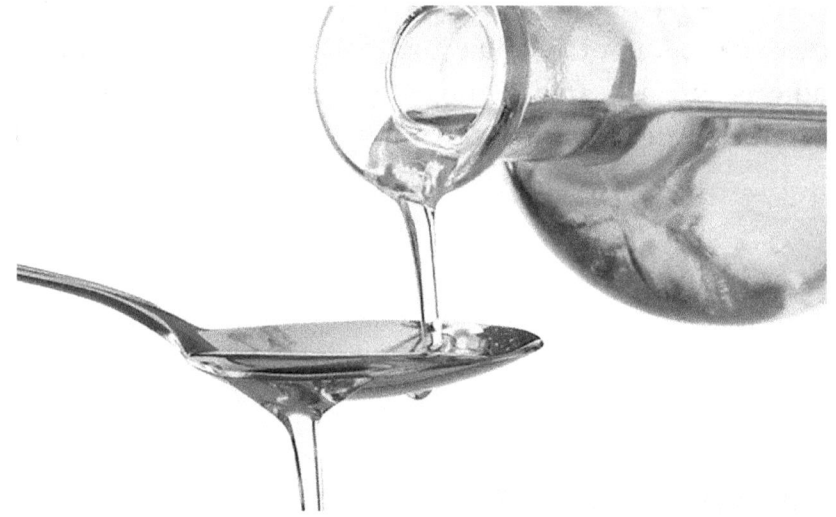

As with other oils, coconut oil contains 100 percent fat. However, it is the type of fat it contains that makes it unique. Most all dietitians know that coconut oil has a high saturated fat content. This makes up about 85 percent of its fatty acids. However, the oil also has about 65 percent of fats that are made up of medium chain acids or MCFA. This is in contrast to long chain fatty acids that are found in other fat sources.

Medium chain fatty acids do not need to break down in the body as single-fatty acids for the body to absorb them. They are capable of going directly through the liver and bypass the carnitine transport system in the body. This is a scientific way of saying that now it is widely known that this oil is extremely healthy for humans and not just as a food, but as a natural beauty product.

It is pure and safe, and it is regarded as one of the healthiest foods a person can enjoy. It should be noted that the healthiest version of the oil is the unrefined version. Organic virgin coconut oil from green coconuts is perfect for healthy cooking. Its many health benefits have been researched and proven to be legitimate.

It might seem very counterintuitive that fat loss can be produced by fat intake. However, coconut oil can play an important role in a balanced weight loss plan. First of all, coconut oil contains 2.6% less calories per gram compared to other fats. Although this 100 calorie per pound of fat difference might seem to be quite small, over time it can be significant.

In March 2008 a study was published in the American Journal of Clinical Nutrition. In the study, 49 overweight women and men adopted a calorie restricted diet (1,800 calories for men, 1,500 calories for women). It included a daily dose of olive oil or MCT oil (24 grams for men, 18 grams for women), which represented 12% of total energy intake over a 16 week period.

Both of the groups of participants lost weight. However, the MCT group had a more significant weight loss. The group consuming olive oil lost 3 pounds, while the group consuming MCT oil lost an average of 7 pounds. The results of the study were in line with some other studies that showed a reduction in body fat and weight in overweight study participants consuming MCT oil.

Coconut oil's MCT fat have a unique structure, which makes it easier to burn them and more difficult to store them in adipose tissues when compared with LCAs that are contained in a majority of other fats, which includes olive oil. Increased energy expenditure and postprandial thermogenesis have been observed in obese as well as lean subjects after ingesting as much as 30 grams of MCT oil or as few as 5 to 10 grams as part of a meal as compared to the identical amount of LCFAs.

In some of the studies, the MCT or coconut oil was hidden in the food in order for the study to be double-blinded. However, it is possible that just substituting the cooking oils and fats that clients commonly use, like margarine and vegetable oils, might facilitate weight loss even more effectively.

Many individuals participating in some weight loss studies that use MCT or coconut oil have also reported more stable energy levels and higher satiety, which can also help with facilitating losing weight.

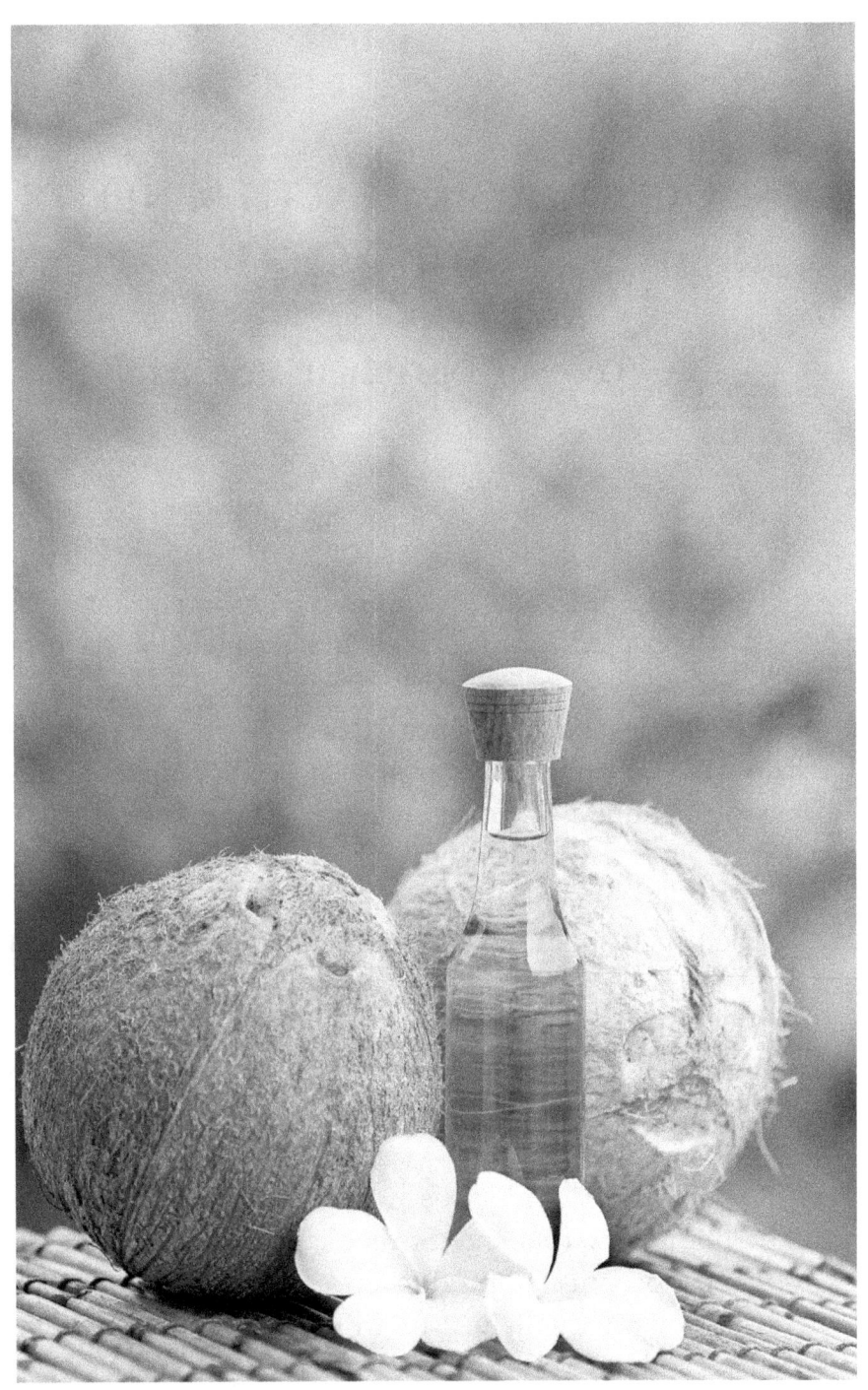

COCONUT OIL HEALTH BENEFITS AND USES

COCONUT OIL HEALTH BENEFITS

Coconut oil provides many important health benefits, including regulating metabolism, proper digestion, boosted immune system, weight loss, cholesterol level maintenance, stress relief, skin care and hair care. It also offers relief from cancer, HIV, diabetes, high blood pressure, heart disease and kidney problems. It also helps to improve bone strength and dental quality.

The benefits that the oil provides can be attributed to the caprylic acid, capric acid and lauric acid contained in the oil, along with their respective properties, like soothing, antibacterial, anti-fungal, antioxidant and antimicrobial qualities.

Coconut oil is widely used in tropical countries such as the Philippines, Thailand, Sri Lanka and India, where there is good coconut oil production. At one point in time, coconut oil was widely used in western countries such as Canada and the United State as well.

However, during the 1970s a strong propaganda campaign was spread against coconut oil by the soy oil and corn oil industry. Due to coconut oil's high saturated fat content, it was considered to be harmful for human bodies until this past decade (2000's) when individuals started questioning the propaganda's claims. Now let's take a closer look at how coconut oil works inside our bodies.

How Our Bodies Use Lauric Acid

Lauric acid is converted into monolaurin by the human body. This supposedly helps with dealing with bacteria and viruses that cause diseases like HIV, cytomegalo virus, influenza and herpes. It also helps with fighting harmful bacteria like helicobacter pylori and listeria monocytogenes, along with giardia lamblia and other harmful protozoa.

Due to the numerous health benefits that coconut oil provides, although the exact action mechanism was not known, it has been widely used in the ancient Indian medicinal system of Ayurveda. A list of possible coconut oil benefits in both modern and traditional medicine has been compiled by the Coconut Research Center.

We need to understand the composition of coconut oil before exploring its benefits.

Coconut Oil Composition

Saturated fats make up over ninety percent of the composition of coconut oil (Don't worry! It isn't nearly as bad as it sounds. Keep reading this entire review to see if your opinion changes), in addition to traces of a couple unsaturated fatty acids. It is the same with virgin coconut oil.

Saturated Fatty Acids

A majority of these are medium chain triglycerides. They supposedly assimilate well within the systems of the body. The chief contributor is lauric acid, which represents over forty percent of the overall total, followed by palmitic, myristic acid, caprylic acid and capric acid.

Monounsaturated Fatty Acid: Oleic Acid

1.   Polyunsaturted fatty acid: Linoleic acid

2.   Poly-phenols: Gallic acid, which is a phenolic acid, is contained in coconut. Polyphenols provide the taste and fragrance of coconut oil. There is a rich amount of these polyphenols in Virgin Coconut Oil.

3.   Certain fatty acid derivatives like polyolesters, monoglycerides, fatty polysorbates, fatty esters, ethoxylates, ethanolamide and betaines.

4.	Fatty alcohol ether sulphate, fatty alcohol sulphate and arty chlorides are all fatty alcohol derivatives.

5.	Vitamin K, vitamin E as well as iron and other minerals.

Hair Care

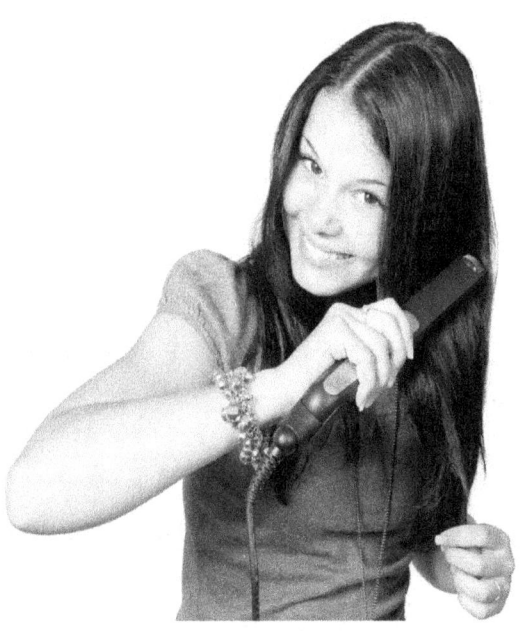

One of the best natural nutrients to use on your hair is coconut oil. It makes your hair shiny and helps with healthy growth of your hair. In addition, it is very effective in reducing the amount of protein loss. Losing too much protein can result in your hair acquiring various unhealthy or unattractive qualities.

Coconut oil is widely used for hair care on the Indian sub-continent. A majority of people living in those countries put coconut oil into their hair on a daily basis after showering or bathing. It is a great conditioner and also helps with damaged hair's re-growth process.

In addition, it provides essential proteins that are needed for healing and nourishing damaged hair. According to several studies, coconut oil offer the hair better protection from damage that hygral fatigue causes.

By using coconut oil to massage your head on a regular basis, it will ensure that your scalp is dandruff-free, even if you have a chronically dry scalp. In addition, it helps to keep your scalp and hair free from lice eggs and lice. Therefore, coconut oil is utilized as hair care oil in addition to being used to manufacture different dandruff relief creams and conditioners. For hair care, coconut oil is usually applied topically.

Heart Diseases \ Cardiovascular Disease

Among many people, there is a big misconception that gets spread around that coconut oil isn't good for the health of your heart. That is because there is a large amount of saturated fats contained in it. However, coconut oil actually benefits the heart. It is comprised of around 50% lauric acid. This helps to actively prevent different heart problems such as high blood pressure and high cholesterol levels. The saturated fats contained in coconut are actually not as harmful as what is in vegetable oils. For example, coconut oil doesn't increase LDL levels, and also reduces damage to arteries and incidence of injury, therefore helping to prevent atherosclerosis.

Despite all of the research, a majority of dieticians are not comfortable recommending that their clients use coconut oil due to the fact that it has high saturated fat content. However, it is important to keep in mind that there is no association of dietary saturated fats with stroke and heart disease, according to the meta-analysis that appeared in the American Journal of Clinical Nutrition's. (Data was examined by researchers from nearly 350,000 individuals. They were then followed up with by as many as 23 years.

The findings of the study showed no relationship between risk of stroke and cardiovascular diseases and saturated fat intake.) Also, the kinds of saturated fats that are in coconut oil actually do have a different structures. This makes it impossible to draw any conclusions by comparing them directly with LCFAs.

In further support of coconut oil's safety, a randomized clinical trial was conducted by researchers where 40 middle-aged Brazilian women that had abdominal obesity were given 2 teaspoons of coconut or soybean oil on a daily basis for 12 weeks. Both groups had lost weight when the study was complete, however just the coconut oil group experienced a significant waist circumference decrease.

For the soybean oil group, there was a significant increase in levels of LDL and total cholesterol, which worsened these individuals cardiovascular risk profiles.

For the women who were part of the coconut oil group, their blood lipid profile didn't significantly change. However, they did have a tendency to have a higher HDL cholesterol level, which indicated improved cardiovascular health. MCTs are not incorporated into chylomicrons so they are more likely to be quickly used for energy.

There have been other studies that have shown decreased inflammatory cytokines, like interleukin-6 (IL-6) and tumor necrosis factor alpha, when MCT oil or coconut oil is consumed.

Some researchers have also seen improved insulin sensitivity for patients who have type 2 diabetes and consume coconut oil. Participants in one study went on a 5 day diet where 40% of calories came from fat and then 77.5% came from either LCFAs or MCTs. Health individuals saw a 17% increase in their insulin sensitivity and individuals with type 2 diabetes saw a 30% increase. The euglycemic clamp technique was used to measure the increase.

Neurological Conditions

According to research, MCT oil can also improve glucose metabolism inside the brain with Alzheimer's disease. It is sometimes called type 3 diabetes since it is associated with glucose metabolism declining inside the brain. That is why dietary strategies promoting ketosis might help the brain with obtaining an alternative energy source. Although glucose has a tendency to be the primary energy source of the brain on the regular high carbohydrate American diet, over half of the energy needs of the brain can be supplied by ketone bodies when glucose and carbohydrates are scarce.

Alzheimer's Disease

There are Alzheimer's disease studies that show how ketone bodies may enhance mitochondrial efficiency as well as make the brain rely less on glucose. In addition to epilepsy, other promising neuroprotective properties that ketone bodies have has been seen in Parkinson's disease and malignant brain cancer.

Dieticians can assist their clients with achieving higher ketone body levels through recommending the adoption of a lower carbohydrate and higher fat diet when it is warranted by their condition.

Using MCT oil or coconut oil can also help with boosting the ketogenic potential of various dietary interventions, since more ketone bodies are produced by MCFAs gram for gram compared to fat that are rich in long-chain triglycerides.

Skin Care

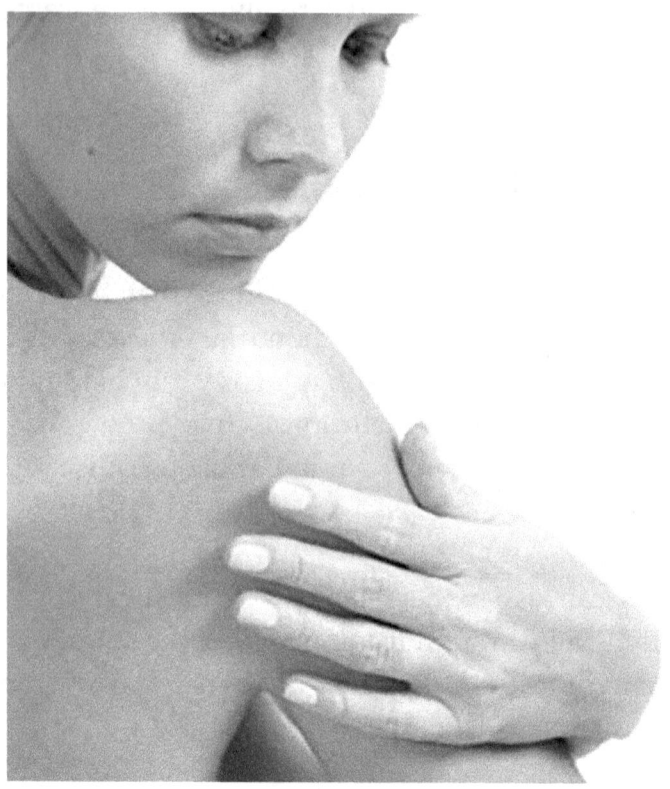

Another benefit of coconut oil is that it is also a great massage oil that can be used on the skin. It is a very effective moisturizer that can be used on all skin types, including dry skin.

The benefits coconut oil provides to the skin are comparable to those that mineral oil provides. Unlike mineral oil however, there isn't any chance of there being adverse side effects to the skin from applying coconut oil. Therefore, it is a safe solution to prevent flaking and dryness of skin. Coconut oil also delays sagging of skin and wrinkles which usually accompany aging.

It also helps to treat numerous skin problems that include eczema, dermatitis, psoriasis and other types of skin infections. That is why coconut oil is a base ingredient in many different body care products such as creams, lotions and soaps used in skin care. In addition, coconut oils helps to prevent degenerative disease and premature aging due to it having well-known antioxidant properties.

Weight Loss

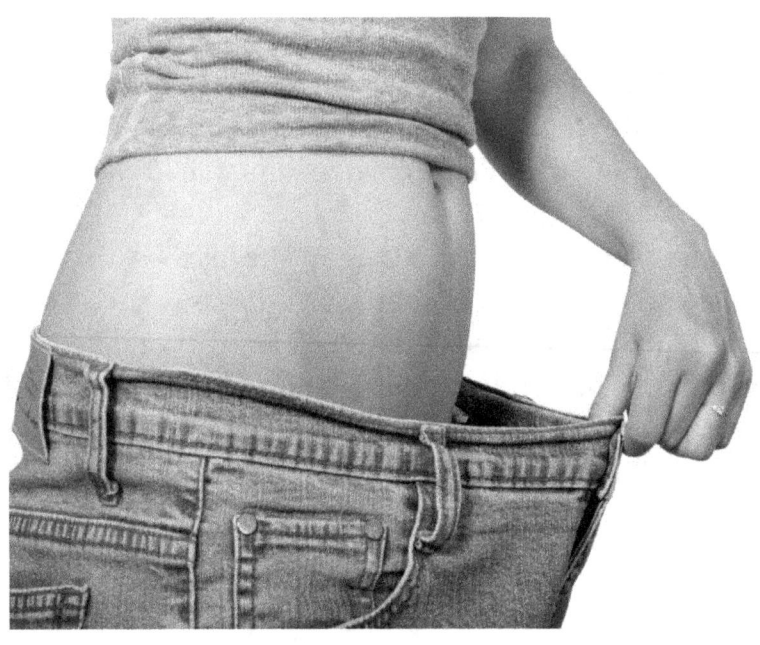

When it comes to losing weight, coconut oil is quite useful. It contains medium and short-chain fatty acids that help with getting rid of excess weight. In addition it digests very easily and also helps with the healthy functioning of the endocrine and thyroid systems. It also helps with increasing the metabolic rate of the body by removing stress from the pancreas, which helps burn more energy and assists overweight and obese individuals with losing weight. Therefore, individuals who reside in tropical coastal regions, who use coconut oil on a daily basis as their main cooking oil, usually are not overweight, obese or fat.

Immunity

In addition, coconut oil benefits the immune system. It strengthens it due to the fact that it contains caprylic acid, capric acid, lauric acid and antimicrobial lipids which have antivial, antibacterial and antifungal properties. Lauric acid is converted into monolaurin by the human body.

Research has supported this as an effective way of dealing with bacteria and viruses that cause diseases such as HIV, cytomegalovirus, influenza and herpes. Coconut oil helps with fighting harmful bacteria such as helicobacter pylori and listeria monocytogenes, as well as harmful protozoa like giardia lamblia.

Digestion

Coconut oil internal functions take place mainly due to the fact that it is used as a cooking oil. When used in this manner, coconut oil helps with improving the digestive system, which helps to prevent various digestion and stomach-related problems such as Irritable Bowel Syndrome. Saturated fats are contained in coconut oil, which have antimicrobial properties that help to deal with various parasites, fungi and bacteria that causes indigestion. In addition, coconut oil helps with absorbing other nutrients like amino acids, minerals and vitamins.

Candida

It has been shown that coconut helps to prevent candida and even cure it. It provides relief from both external and internal inflammation that candida causes. It has the capacity for retaining high moisture, which prevents the skin from peeling off or cracking.

In addition, unlike other candida pharmaceutical treatments, coconut oil effects are gradual and not sudden or drastic, which gives a patient plenty of time to grow accustomed to Herxheimer Reactions (symptoms that accompany the body rejecting toxins that are generated as these fungi are eliminated) or withdrawal symptoms.

However, when this condition is treated, individuals should gradually and systematically increase their coconut oil dosages and shouldn't initially start with a big quantity.

Candida, or Systemic Candidiasis as it is also called, is a serious disease that is caused by an uncontrolled and excessive growth of the yeast known as Candida Albicans inside the stomach. The yeast is inside everyone's stomach to a certain extent. However, no adverse effects are manifested since beneficial bacterial also residing in the stomach controls it growth.

There are numerous reasons for uncontrolled yeast growth. If there are other destructive bacteria or antibiotics used which eliminate these bacteria, the bacteria can become imbalanced, which can result in a problem such as Candida developing. In addition, bleaching or washing the stomach with excessive amounts of chemical laxatives or medicine or ingesting poisonous materials can cause fungi or yeast to begin to grow rapidly and result in Candida.

Candida Symptoms

These include infections in the throat, nose, ear, intestines, stomach, bladder, urinary tract and genitals, dry and itchy skin, inflammations in the skin and internal organs, peeling off and patching of skin (especially in the scalp), excretory and digestive disorders and nail and hair problems.

The disease is quite common in America and Europe, maybe due to the moist and cold climate and the way food is prepared, stored and consumed. In these areas, much of the food is processed in one or another with yeast or is fermented.

As an example, those cultures rely heavily on foods such as bread as well as other types of baked goods, cheese and wine and other types of alcoholic beverages. These things also help with Candida Albicans growing inside the body. The different fatty acids that are in coconut oil help to counteract the effects of those habits and also can be used for treating Candida.

Capric Acid

Capric Acid is a type of saturated fat (medium chain fatty acid) that is contained in coconut oil. It has antifungal, antiviral and antimicrobial properties. This fatty acid is also contained in breast milk. It protects an infant from fungal, viral and bacterial infections.

Inside the body, capric acid reacts with specific enzymes that other bacteria secretions. This converts it subsequently into a potent antimicrobial agent called monocaprin. In using coconut oil systematically for treating Candida, it has also been found that capric acid is very effective at killing yeast.

Lauric acid, myristic acid, caproic acid and caprylic acid are all in coconut oil. They have antifungal and antimicrobial properties which help with eliminating candida albicans. The medium chain fatty acid and saturated fat lauric acid forms a compound that is called monolaurin whenever it reacts with enzymes. Monolaurin is a very powerful fungus and germ killer.

Healing Wounds and Getting Rid Of Infections

When coconut oil is applied in a wound or an infected area, it forms a layer that offers protection the wound from air, bacteria, fungi, viruses and any dust. Apart from this benefit, coconut oil makes the process of healing faster. Therefore the wound closes up faster and heals in the right way.

Coconut has properties that fight fungi, viruses and bacteria.in relation to the findings of The Coconut Research Centre, coconut combats all the viruses that are common. These includes those that cause measles, hepatitis, SARS, influenza, herpes and any other common viruses that can affect the health of a person.

It also gets rids of bacteria that is responsible or infections such as gonorrhea, urinary tract infection and ulcers. Coconut oil also kills fungi that cause ringworms, diaper rush and thrush.

COCONUT NUTRITIONAL VALUE

Product	Definition	Nutritional Value	Use
Coconut oil	Oil extracted from coconut meat	100% fat	Excellent for cooking and baking
Coconut water	Liquid found inside young coconuts	Natural sugars and electrolytes combined with only traces of protein and fat	Great postworkout drink
Coconut milk	Liquid obtained from pressing grated coconut meat	Dairy- and lactose-free milk that's rich in fats	Dairy-free alternative for smoothies, creamy sauces, and soups
Coconut cream	Same as coconut milk, only with less water (thicker consistency)	Higher in fat compared with coconut milk	
Coconut flour	Ground dried, defatted coconut meat	Low in carbohydrates and rich in fiber	Cookies, muffins, and other baked goods (requires special recipes and can't replace other flours using a simple ratio)
Coconut butter	Ground coconut meat with the consistency of a nut butter	High in fat (also known as coconut manna or coconut cream concentrate)	Can be used as any nut butter: by the spoonful, as a spread, in smoothies, or in baked goods recipes

VARIETIES OF COCONUT OIL

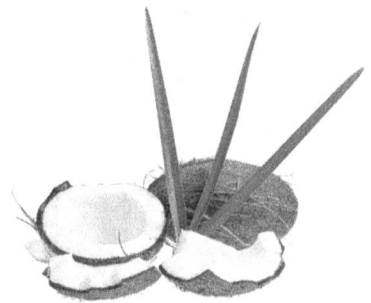

There are many varieties of coconut oil. The six that are available in the market include refined oil, pure oil, virgin oil, organic oil, extra virgin oil and organic virgin oil.

Refined Oil

Refined oil is sometimes known as RBD coconut oil. It is coconut oil that is different from the usual because it has been bleached, deodorized and refined. In reference to its name, this type of coconut oil is made by technical and chemical bleaching, refining and deodorizing raw and unrefined coconut oil. This process results in coconut oil that is colorless, thin and odorless. In addition to this, it does not have any suspension of particles in it. It is a pure form of started fats.

Pure Oil

Pure oil is what is used by most people. It is a clean and very natural kind of coconut oil.it is formed from copra, which refers to coconut kernels that have been dried out. It does not contain any form of artificial additives. The extraction takes place by using a compressing mill on the copra. This mill is powered using electricity or bullocks. The type of oil extracted by bullock is considered to be better. It is used for massaging, in hair, the cosmetic industry and as medicine.

Virgin Oil

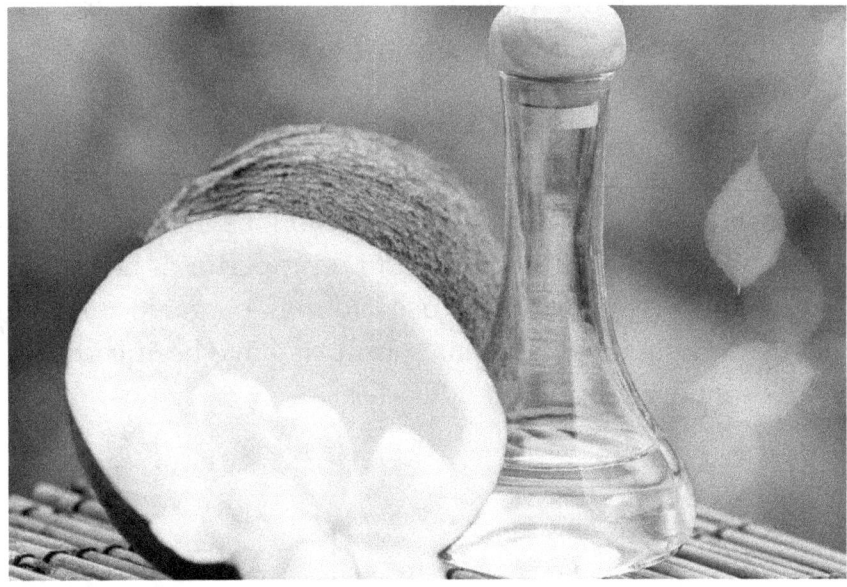

Virgin oil is derived from is extracted from coconut flesh. This is by use of the milk contained in the coconut meat. Contrary to pure coconut milk which is derived from copra, virgin oil is extracted through the process of both centrifugal separation, fermentation and the actions of enzymes. This process involves the use of little or no heat. This is to ensure that the oil maintains its natural fatty acids as well as antioxidants. It is a preferred form of coconut oil.

Organic Oil

Organic oil is a form of coconut oil that is extracted from coconuts. However these coconuts are straight from coconut palms. The palms are grown in soil that contains only natural and organic manure. This soil does not have any insecticides or artificial fertilizer in them. This organic oil is made even more natural by the fact that the extraction process does not involve any artificial additives.

For this reason, organic oil is a major ingredient in most cosmetic products. These include the organic creams, organic soaps and organic body lotions that are used to enhance beauty due to the natural properties it has. Organic oil is also edible and it is used to make organic snacks and other edible foods. Organic products have been certified by relevant organizations and bodies.

Organic Virgin Coconut Oil

Organic virgin coconut oil simply refers to virgin coconut oil that has been organically extracted from organic coconut. It is a very rare form of virgin coconut oil which contains all the antioxidant properties. It is a highly preferred version of coconut oil due to its high content of organic properties.

Extra Virgin Oil

Extra virgin oil is a highly questionable form of coconut oil. This is because it is very difficult to understand the name of this kind of coconut oil. The fact that there are no official levels of virginity for oil. It is hard to tell the degree of virginity of oil. The government and other large companies have not commented on extra virgin oil and its acceptability. This means that this oil has to be researched on further.

Coconut oils of different varieties have more or less similar properties. Before one purchases any of the coconut oil varieties, they need to do some research so as to determine the variety that satisfies what they are looking for.

Coconut oil can be used effectively as a carrier oil. Carrier oil has a range of uses. It is a highly respected oil when it comes to Chinese medicine, aromatherapy, Ayurveda and other types of therapy and treatment that constitute massaging. Carrier oils are preferred because they are quickly and easily seeped into the skin. If used in conjunction with other oils, it enhances their absorption into the skin. It can also be added to herbal extracts.

In addition to this, coconut oil does not become rancid. It cannot be overpowered by other oils, medicines and herbal extracts when it is mixed with them. This is because it is a very stable oil. It therefore keeps the oils it is mixed with protected from bacteria and fungi. It maintains the contents and properties of the oils and herbs mixed with it. Coconut can however be very costly in some countries. It is affordable in tropical countries.

SOME OTHER GREAT BENEFITS OF COCONUT OIL

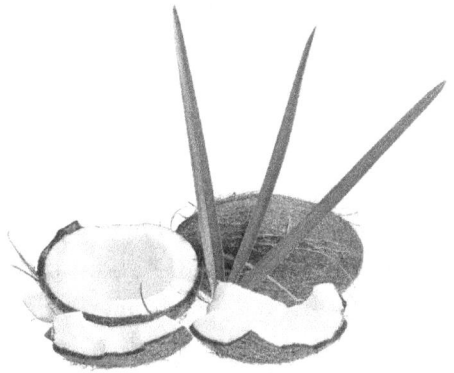

It is highly recommended that coconut oil be used for numerous other benefits that are detailed below. The following have been shown to be mildly helped by using coconut oil:

Liver:

Coconut oil contains fatty acids and medium chain triglycerides which help to prevent liver disease since those substances are converted into energy easily when they get to the liver. This reduces the liver's work load and helps to prevent fat accumulation as well.

Kidney:

Using coconut oil helps to prevent gall bladder and kidney diseases. In addition, it helps with dissolving kidney stones.

Pancreatitis:

It is believed that coconut oil helps to treat pancreatitis.

Stress Relief:

One characteristic of coconut oil is that it is very soothing, and therefore helps with removing stress. To eliminate or reduce mental fatigue, apply some coconut oil to your head and then have a gentle massage.

Diabetes:

Using coconut oil can help with improving secretion of insulin and controlling blood sugar. Utilizing blood glucose effectively is also promoted, which helps to prevent and treat diabetes.

Bones:

As previously mentioned, coconut oil helps to improve our body's ability to absorb essential minerals. They include magnesium and calcium, which are both necessary for bone development. Therefore, coconut oil is quite useful for women prone to osteoporosis once they get past middle age.

Dental Care:

One important component of teeth is calcium. Coconut oil helps the body absorb calcium, so it is helpful with developing strong teeth and also helps to stop tooth decay.

Cancer And HIV:

Coconut oil is thought to play an important role in reducing an individual's viral susceptibility to HIV in cancer patients. There is preliminary research that indicates that this effect that coconut oil has reduces HIV patients' viral load.

Coconut oil is also frequently used by dieters, body builders and athletes. This is because there are fewer calories contained in coconut oil than other oils. It also doesn't lead to fat accumulation in the arteries and heart and is converted into energy easily. Coconut oil enhances athletic performance and boosts endurance and energy.

WHY COCONUT OIL IS SOLID

Coconut oil, unlike a majority of other oils, has a high melting point of around 76-78 degrees Fahrenheit or 24-25 degrees Celsius. Therefore, at room temperature it is solid and only melts when the temperature is considerably higher. So, if you purchase a bottle of coconut oil that is solid, you don't need to assume it has a problem. Coconut oil is frequently in solid form, and you don't need to keep it inside the refrigerator.

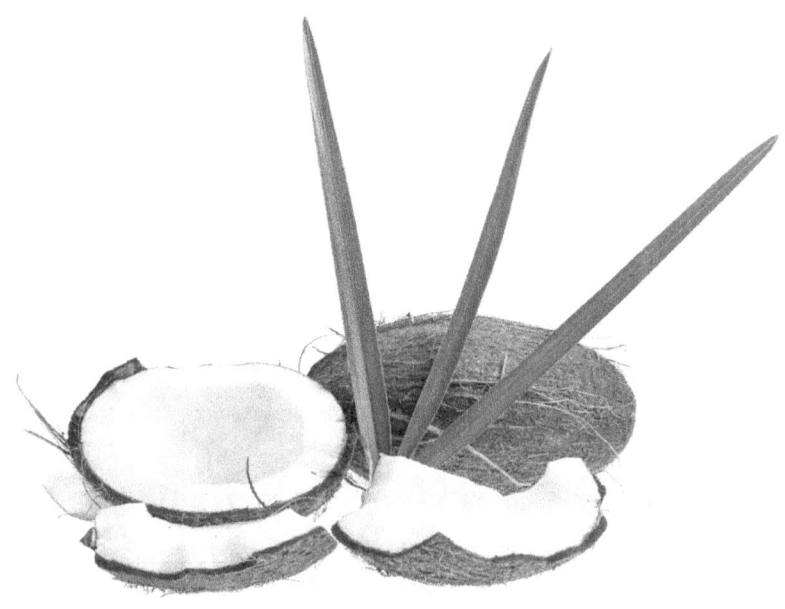

HOW TO USE COCONUT OIL

When coconut oil is used for topical purposes, particularly for hair care, if the oil is solid just melt it by soaking the bottle in warm water or placing it in the sun. Some coconut oil can also be placed into a small bowl and then the bowl can be heated over a flame (however, don't put inside a microwave). The oil can then be placed in your palm and applied to your hair.

For internal consumption, just replace vegetable oils or butter in your recipes with coconut oil. Keep in mind, it isn't necessary for you to switch completely to coconut oil, since you will lose benefits from dairy products and more traditional oils. Can coconut oil be used for cooking? Yes, coconut oil is used for cooking by people in most tropical coastal areas.

I DON'T LIKE THE TASTE OF COCONUT OIL

So what should I do? You can try to use coconut oil in various types of recipes to see if it appeals to you in different dishes. However, if after consuming coconut oil you get nauseated, don't force yourself. Like with any item of food, your body could be allergic possibly to coconut oil so it is better to not eat it.

HOW TO BUY COCONUT OIL

There are many varieties of coconut oil. Some are designed for specific uses. The first step in deciding which type of coconut oil to purchase is to clearly define why one needs the oil. In addition to this, know the specific place that the coconut oil will be used. For instance, the coconut oil could be used for massage, aromatherapy, in food or even as a form of medicine. Although there is a variety of coconut oil forms, they vary in very minimal ways.

There are a number of reasons as to why one may purchase coconut oil. The many types of coconut oil are made to serve various purposes. Cooking can be done by refined oil. Weight loss is most effective when one uses the virgin form of coconut oil. When coconut oil is taken up as a carrier, the forms that are most effective are virgin as well as fractionated oil.

Coconut oil that is effective for massage and aromatherapy are the pure and refined versions. Pure as well as refined forms of coconut oil are better used for hair to make it soft and shiny. For the purpose of healing wounds and other medicinal purposes, virgin or virgin organic forms of coconut oil can be used.

The preferred edible form of coconut oil is virgin and organic. This is because it retains its natural properties during extraction. Coconut oil that has been refined is very hygienic and has no contamination.

The forms of coconut oil that is easily accessible to users

in stores is the pure and the refined versions. The availability of these oils in tropical areas is much more than in other parts of the world. Some varieties such as virgin and organic oil are not easily found in stores. However, they may be found in large and well supplied drug stores and general stores.

Countries that do not have the ability to produce coconut oil may find it challenging to have the various forms of oil at their reach. This is mostly the case for Canada, US and some sections of Europe. Coconut oil varieties are mostly found in highly populated countries such as Philippines, Thailand, Coastal Africa, Sri Lanka and India. It would therefore be advisable to use online methods to order any rare types of coconut oil that one may want to buy.

There are many brands of coconut oil available in the market. In most rural areas, it may be normal to find that coconut oil is manually produced by local inhabitants. It may be good to purchase such coconut oil if the person extracting it is hygienic and does it the right way. Other than this, it is advisable to purchase coconut oil that is reputable and trusted in the market. Ensure that the manufacturing and expiry date as well as the ingredients of the oil are well explained.

As soon as one buys coconut oil, storage is a key factor to ensure that its properties are maintained. It is best stored in broad containers for users in cold countries. Ensure that the containers lid can be tightly sealed. The tin should have a broad mouth to enable one to easily scoop oil from it. The container should be sealed whenever the oil is not in use to ensure that it is not contaminated by dust and insects.

LET'S LOOK AT HOW YOU CAN PUT COCONUT OIL TO USE

COOKING..USE REFINED COCONUT OIL

AS A CARRIER OIL......................................VIRGIN COCONUT OIL - FRACTIONATED COCONUT OIL

WEIGHT LOSS..USE VIRGIN COCONUT OIL

OVERALL HEALTH...................................ORGANIC COCONUT OIL - VIRGIN COCONUT OIL

MEDICINAL USES...............................VIRGIN ORGANIC COCONUT OIL - VIRGIN COCONUT OIL

HAIR CARE...REFINED COCONUT OIL - PURE COCONUT OIL

BODY MASSAGE................................ REFINED COCONUT OIL - PURE COCONUT OIL

COCONUT WATER HEALTH BENEFITS AND USES

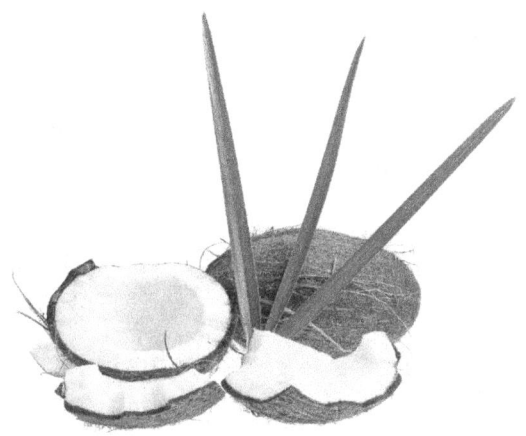

The water found in coconuts is great to use topically and also in recipes and simply by itself as a treatment for many conditions, as well as providing an array of benefits. For example, it is very hydrating, it can help you lower your cholesterol and this oil can also help with certain digestive disorders, among other things. Coconut palm trees have long been regarded as producing a fruit that has helped people in many ways. It's not just the coconut but the entire tree itself that has uses, too. Inside a coconut is the coconut oil or water and of course the coconut flesh. All parts of the coconut have important nutrients that provide your body with the right nourishment and also boost energy levels naturally. As mentioned, the coconut comes from a palm tree, and Cocos Nucifera is its scientific name. While many think of a coconut simply being a 'nut,' it is known as a fruit.

The origin of the coconut tree is believed to have stemmed from Asia, but it wasn't long before coconuts had made it to both Europe and Africa. You can find palm tree varieties just about anywhere that harbors a tropical climate these days. Not every palm variety produces the coconut, but the coconut trees are numerous in many areas. Within the country of India, people have been using coconuts for various reasons for centuries.

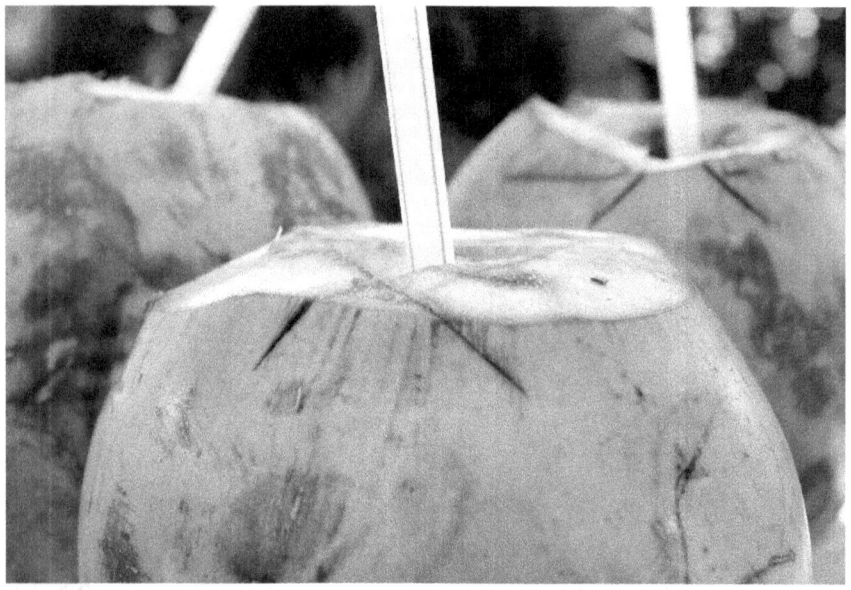

They aren't just used for bodily health benefits and treatment for conditions but also for offerings of gratitude to the gods. The Sanskrit language translates the coconut tree into a tree that grants wishes to people. The reason behind this meaning is that there are so many useful parts of the tree for all kinds of beneficial reasons.

A coconut can be up to 30 centimeters long, and it's said to be like a rugby ball in reference to its shape and size. Coconut shells are extremely hard, and each coconut has what is known as 'coir,' which is the fibrous layers covering the coconut. Inside the hard coconut shell is the flesh of the coconut and the coconut water. When it comes to products associated with coconuts, you have coconut milk, wine, oil and much more, so the water and coconut flesh or meat help to make many things.

As for the benefits of the water found in coconuts, a person gets dietary fiber, extra energy, healthy fats and carbohydrates and much more. As for the minerals and vitamins contained in the rest of the coconut, the list goes on and on. You are going to be blown away when you see that coconut is a good source of potassium, iron, vitamin B6, folate, magnesium and that's just for starters! There are so many more nutrients contained in coconuts, and that is why they are used for so many different things.

Some Of The Great Health Benefits Of Coconut Water

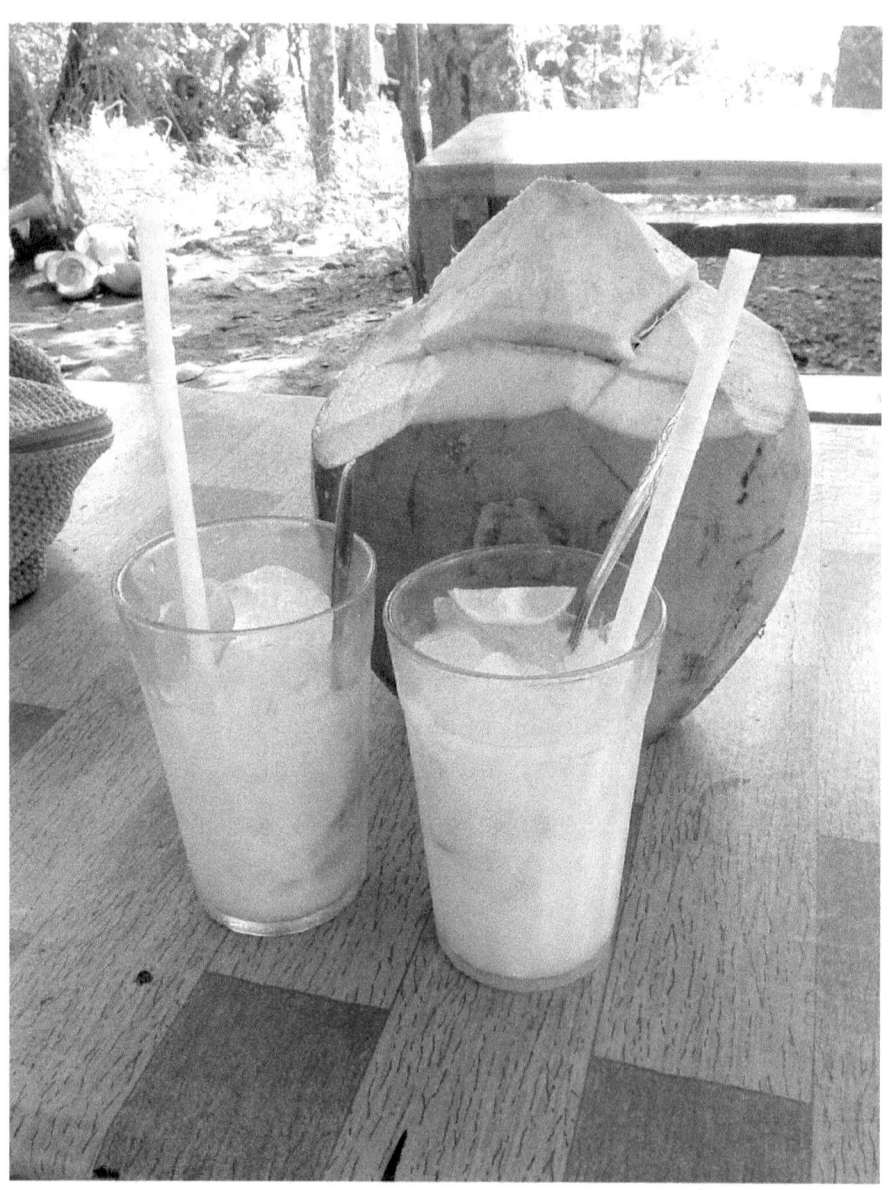

The following are some of the health benefits that come from drinking coconut water:

Re-hydrates The Body:

Coconut water isn't only water. This water is full of minerals and vitamins. Some minerals contained in coconut water, like sodium and potassium, act as electrolytes, which helps with balancing the water levels inside our bodies. Drinking a glass or two of coconut water after being out in the sun all day can help to restore lost energy, vitamins and minerals very quickly.

Helps With Digestive System Disorders:

Flatulence, dyspepsia, dysentery, mild diarrhea, vomiting and gastroenteritis can all be helped by coconut water. Research studies have shown that coconut water makes for a great home remedy for children with mild diarrhea.

Helps with Intravenous Hydration:

You can also use coconut water for resuscitation and intravenous hydration for patients who are seriously ill when there are no regular intravenous hydration solutions available.

Note: Medical professionals are the only ones who are experienced and capable enough to administer it. Don't try doing this at home on your own.

Antimicrobial Properties:

Tests have been conducted on the antimicrobial properties of coconut water. Coconut water contains peptides, which is a biochemical that can kill gram negative and gram positive bacteria. Therefore, it can be very helpful to drink coconut water to fight infections.

Benefits Cholera:

Tender coconut water can help if you are suffering from cholera. Mix 3 or 4 tablespoons lime juice with two glass full of coconut water. This solution will help to bring the electrolyte balance back. The patient should be given this solution regularly. Coconut water is a good potassium source, which can be the perfect cholera solution.

Controls Cholesterol:

Another benefit of coconut water is that it can help to deter high cholesterol. There have been studies that have looked at coconut water's impact on cholesterol-fed rats. It showed that their bad cholesterol levels (LDL or low density lipoprotein) triglycerides and total overall cholesterol levels went down while good cholesterol (HDL or high density lipoprotein) increased after consuming coconut water.

Heart Health:

Coconut water is healthy for the heart. It helps to control cholesterol, so the aorta and heart have lower cholesterol levels. This results in a heart that is healthier with reduced chances for heart attacks and strokes. Coconut water stimulates enzymes. This helps with myocardial damage recovery.

Controls Hypertension:

Coconut water also helps to control high blood pressure (hypertension). A study comparing mauby (popular Caribbean island tree bark-based beverage) and coconut water showed that when hypertensive patients drank coconut water, it showed a greater positive response compared to those given mauby. Drinking tender coconut water every day in the amount of one to two glasses can help to control hypertension.

Good for Liver:

Tender coconut water tests for hepato-protective properties indicates it benefits the liver. It provides antioxidants, which helps to reduce toxin activity inside the liver.

Urinary Disorders:

The diuretic properties of coconut water helps with urinary disorder cases. Because of this diuretic effect, it is easy to expel water from out of the body, in addition to harmful toxins. This helps to keep the bodily systems health and clear of toxins.

Antioxidant Properties:

Antioxidants help with scavenging various toxins and free radicals that are produced naturally inside the body.

Coconut water is an excellent antioxidant source. The free radical may start out with what is referred to as chain reactions inside the body by taking away electrons. These chain reactions may cause cell death along with various other diseases. Antioxidants that are in food are critical to counteracting free radicals, which are dangerous and very unhealthy.

Estrogen-like Hormone Supply:

There have been research studies conducted that show that young coconut water can benefit hormone replacement therapy or postmenopausal symptoms. Coconut water has some wound healing properties as well.

COCONUT OIL FOR HAIR CARE

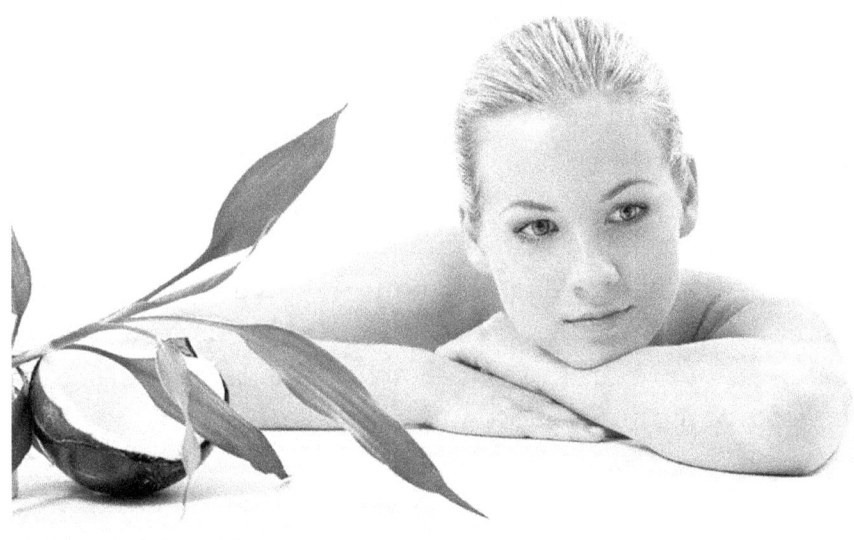

As mentioned above coconut oil is very popular and is frequently used as a form of hair oil. Before you begin to use coconut oil, make sure you read the above to understand why it's so special and why so many people have selected it as their daily hair oil.

Today, many people are residing in coastal regions where coconuts tend to grow in abundance. They already know how sweet the coconuts smell and how the oil is great for many uses. Areas like Sri Lanka, Malaysia, Indonesia,

Burma, The Philippines and other areas in the Caribbean already know how great coconuts are for not just eating, but also for hair and body care.

Rich in carbohydrates as well as vitamins and minerals that are ideal for the body, the uses are as varied as the areas that the coconut is located in. The coconut is used in soaps, cosmetics and even creams worldwide. It's also ideal to eat in salads and other delicious dishes. Anyone that has ever had fresh coconut over the store bought flaked coconut will tell you that there is a huge difference in flavor and consistency.

For many centuries coconut oil has been used on the hair. It keeps the hair strong and nourished and it protects the hair shafts from aging prematurely. It also helps to relieve baldness and hair loss. Here are just a few of the great benefits of the mighty coconut:

EVERYDAY HAIR CARE:

Hair Loss Prevention

Coconut oil is one of the best uses for hair loss prevention. Since ancient times those residing in India and surrounding areas have used coconut oil to prevent hair loss. One remedy involves boiling sage leaves in coconut oil and applying it to the scalp for hair loss prevention.

Lime Water And Coconut Oil

Lime water and coconut oil can help to relieve hair loss as well. Gooseberries mixed with coconut oil are also said to help relieve hair loss. Simply boil the gooseberries in the oil and apply to the hair as a tonic. Leave in for a few minutes or overnight and then wash out just as you would shampoo your hair. Your locks will be lustrous and soft.

Damaged Hair

Damaged hair is no issue if you apply some coconut oil to it. It helps to maintain protein and since its rich in lauric acid it can readily penetrate the hair shaft. This is due to the low molecular weight. It's ideal as a pre wash and as a post wash hair care aid. Anytime your hair is feeling dry or doesn't seem to be doing what it should, try applying some coconut oil to it and see amazing results.

Sweat

If you sweat a lot you may wish to try some coconut oil on your scalp to help cool your head down. It's very soothing and for anyone who suffers from scalp sweating it is an ideal remedy. Simply rub some into the scalp and feel an instant cooling sensation.

Moisturizing

Moisture is important in hair care and coconut oil has many great moisture retaining capabilities. It's not easy to break down nor does it evaporate. Therefore it's very stable and will prevent moisture loss. It helps maintain the integrity of the hair shaft and will prevent breakage.

Conditioner

As a conditioner it's ideal. Far superior to any other conditioner on the market today. It helps to prevent hair loss, keep hair shimmery soft and will soothe an irritated scalp. Stop wasting money on high priced hair care products and buy a jar of coconut oil and you'll see amazing results.

Dandruff

If you're suffering from dandruff, the fatty acids will help to prevent dandruff. Simply apply it to your scalp with some warm water and castor oil and you'll have the best ever dandruff remedy.

Coconut Oil and Sesame Oil

Another way to use it is to make a mix of coconut oil and sesame oil and slather it on the head for about 30 minutes. Shampoo hair as usual and you'll have gorgeous soft shimmery tresses.

Styling Oil

As a styling oil it is unsurpassed. Melting with heat (this can be done by simply allowing it to melt in the hands) and it will protect the hair shaft and when it cools it will condense. Thus, you'll have a thin coat of coconut oil protecting your hair and scalp at all times. It's not heavy or oily feeling and will give you a soothing feeling.

Head Lice

If you've ever battled lice you know well how frustrating it can be. Simply apply some coconut oil to the head and then comb with the fine tooth comb to rid the hair shaft of nits. It will help loosen the nits and suffocate them at the same time thus helping in the prevention of the little critters.

Dry Hair

When it comes to dry hair the coconut oil will help to condition and reduce dry hair issues. No more breakage and no more dull hair. Use it as a soothing oil or cream and watch your dry hair turn gorgeous.

Toning

Toning is no issue when you use coconut oil. Apply it with some essential lavender oil and allow it to sit on the hair and scalp overnight. Then, simply wash it out in the morning and you'll see improved results. Coconut oil just may be the miracle cure for all hair issues.

Soothing Conditioner

One of the best ways to use coconut oil is as a soothing

conditioner to the hair and scalp. If you've recently had any emotional trauma and your hair is breaking off you can simply apply coconut oil and it will soothe the scalp and hair shaft and help to restore hair to its original shine and glow. Perhaps coconut oil is a miracle hair tonic.

Boils

Many people end up with boils on their scalp and this is especially true during the winter months, but this can also be caused by heat or sun exposure. You need to keep your scalp and hair clean, and when you use a mixture of coconut oil and olive oil, and massage them into the hair, then you may get relief from boils. However, if this problem doesn't go away, then you should consider seeing your doctor as soon as possible.

Split Ends

Coconut oil and almond oil can help minimize split ends. Sure, you may want to cut them off, which you should do if you do have a lot of them, but if you notice that it is only a small issue, then try using coconut oil and almond oil. You might be surprised at how well this mixture works.

Baldness And Gray Hair

Coconut oil can also play a role in preventing baldness. It is also thought to be good at preventing gray hair. Here is a tip though. Mix Eclipta Alba leaf juice into coconut oil and then put it on your hair and scalp.

IT IS WIDELY AVAILABLE

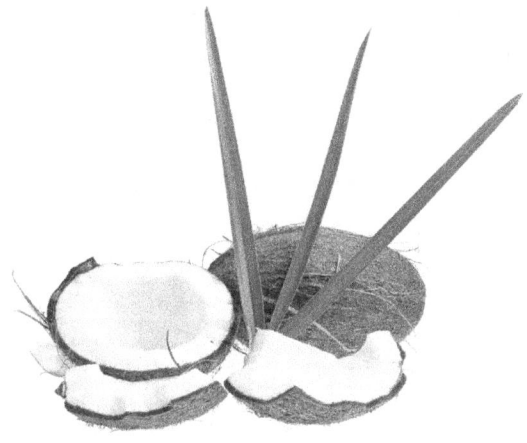

You can find coconut oil in many places and it comes in quite a few different forms. Many use odorless coconut oil, but they still reap the benefits it offers. Also, let's not forget that coconut oil is found in some shampoos.

As a matter of fact, many shampoos contain small amounts of the oil. More and more people are starting to realize just how important some oils are for their hair. Many years ago people really didn't think of using oils in their hair, but times have changed.

If you want your hair to look more natural, then consider using shampoo with coconut oil in it. Also, you may want to consider switching to a coconut oil-based shampoo if you use regular shampoo excessively. If you do this, you may feel and see a difference in your hair as time goes on.

As previously mentioned, many shampoos contain coconut oil, even if it is just a small amount. Many manufacturers have learnt that many men and women want healthy looking hair and that is one of the reasons some manufacturers may choose to use coconut oil in their products.

Plus, don't forget that many people have used coconut oil in their hair for many years, even before it became extremely popular.

Healthy Hair

You could end up seeing some great results if you use coconut oil for your hair, and this is because coconut oil can leave your hair nourished. Not only that, but it has anti-aging properties, as well as provide your hair with moisture. When it comes to keeping the hair healthy, it appears that coconut oil works great.

The Oily Cause

Your hair may feel dry, hard, rough or even bleached if you use soap-based shampoos or detergents. This is why sometimes your comb doesn't go smoothly through the hair, after you have washed it. Coconut oil is derived from natural fats, and the oil can keep your hair shiny and smooth.

Fragrance

Shampoos that contain coconut oil smell great. This is an added bonus. After you wash your hair with coconut oil, you will likely smell a nice scent. If your current shampoo doesn't have coconut oil in it, then add some to it. All you need to do is take some coconut oil and mix it with your current shampoo. If you do this, then you will experience the benefits that coconut oil offers you.

Asides from the things mentioned above, there are other things that you should do if you want to keep your hair looking good and feeling good. Some of these things include keeping your hair clean, as well as eat well and use grooming products. Also, make sure you use a good comb. If you do all of these things, then you will be doing something great for your hair, so start doing those things soon.

Breakfast Recipes

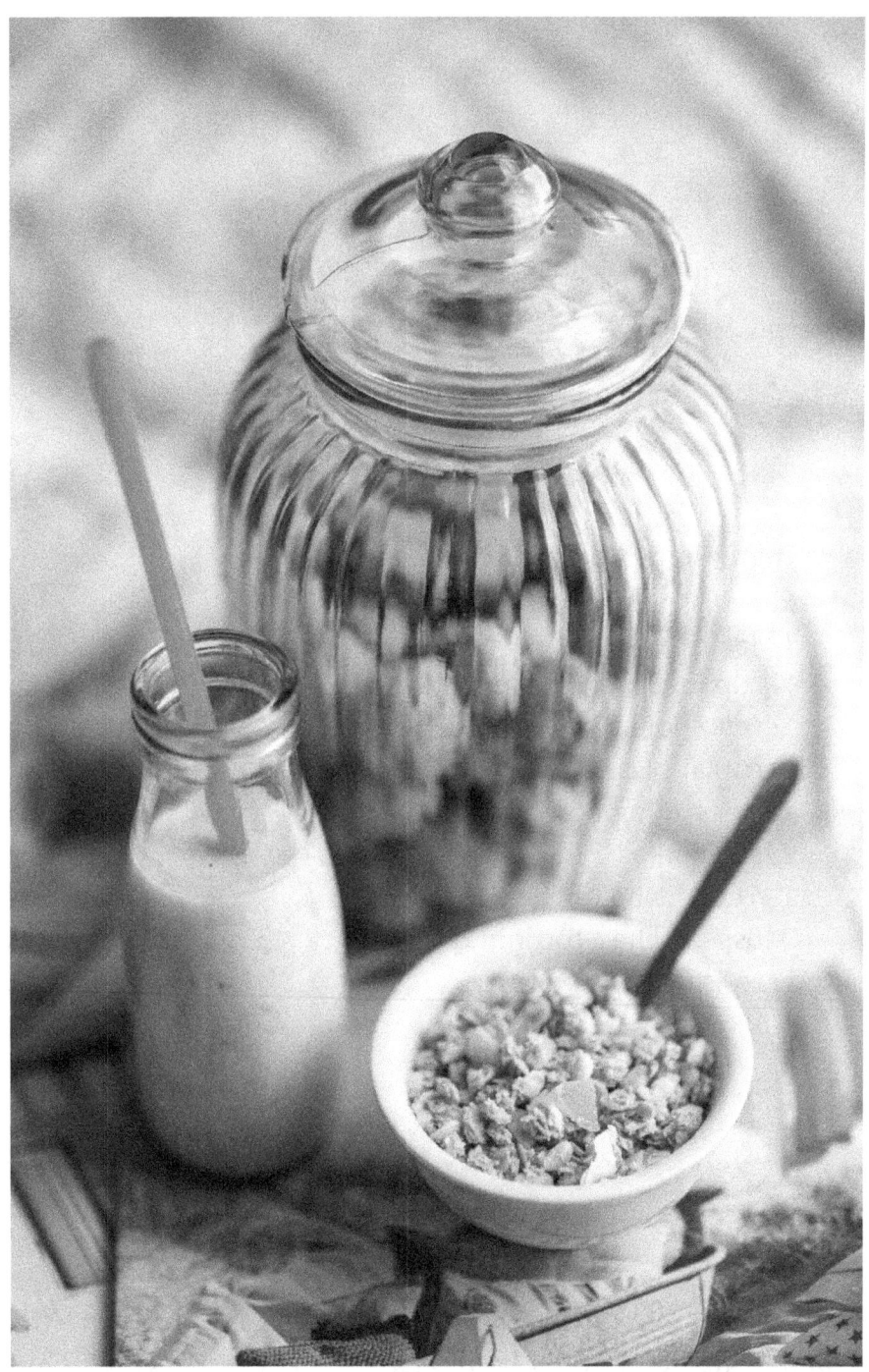

Whole-Wheat Muffins

Makes 12 Muffins

Ingredients You Will Need

1 egg
¾ cup lukewarm water
1/3 cup honey
½ cup applesauce
2 tsps. baking powder
1 tsp vanilla
1 ¾ cups whole-wheat flour
3 tbsps. melted coconut oil
½ tsp salt

Directions

Set the oven to 400 degrees F. and leave to preheat. Mix and combine thoroughly in a large bowl the melted coconut oil, honey, water, vanilla, egg, and applesauce.

Next:

Add to a separate, small bowl the baking powder, flour and salt and mix with a fork. Now, add the dry ingredients to the wet ingredients. Mix until moistened.

Next:

Pour the mixture into the greased muffin cups. Place the cups inside the hot oven and allow to bake for about 15 minutes.

Fluffy Coconut Waffles And Pancakes

Makes 7 – 8 Pancakes

Per Serving: Calories: 146 - Fat: 129 - Protein: 49

Ingredients You Will Need

1 tsp baking powder
3 eggs
2 tsps. Coconut sugar
¾ cup coconut milk
½ cup coconut flour, sifted
3 tbsps. Virgin coconut oil, melted
½ tsp sea salt

Directions

Add to a large bowl the coconut milk, eggs, 2 tablespoons of coconut oil, sugar and salt. Mix well. In a separate small bowl, combine with a spoon the baking powder and coconut flour; and then mix it into the batter until the batter thickens.

Next:

Melt the remaining tablespoon of coconut oil in a skillet at medium heat. Using ¼ cup measuring cup for each pancake; carefully scoop the batter onto skillet.

Cook the pancake for one minute and turn on the opposite side. Cook until pancakes are cooked through or golden brown.

To make the waffles, scoop batter into a well-oiled waffle iron and follow cooking directions on the packet. Pour the coconut pancake syrup on top and serve.

Banana and Coconut Breakfast Muffins

Makes 12 Muffins

Per Serving: Calories: 151 - Fat: 9g - Protein: 4g

Ingredients You Will Need

4 eggs
½ cup nuts, soaked and dehydrated
2-3 ripe bananas, mashed
½ tsp baking powder
½ cup coconut flour
¼ cup coconut oil
¼ cup honey
¼ tsp sea salt

Directions

Set the oven to 350 degrees F. and leave to preheat. Greased muffin pan and set aside. Add to a bowl all the ingredients and mix. Now, scoop the ingredients into the muffin pan. Place inside the oven and allow to bake for 15 minutes or until tan. Serve warm and enjoy.

Pancake Syrup

Per Serving: Calories: 100 - Fat: 59 - Protein: 19

Ingredients You Will Need

1 tsp vanilla extract
1 cup coconut sugar
1 tsp potato starch flour
1 can coconut milk
2 tbsps. Desiccated coconut
2 tsps. filtered water

Directions

Add to a medium size sauce pan the sugar and coconut milk. Mix until the sugar is dissolved. Place the saucepan over medium heat and bring to a boil. Lower the heat to a simmer, always stirring, to prevent syrup from burning.

Mix in a small bowl the potato starch with two teaspoons water. Pour into the syrup mixture, stirring as you pour.

Bring to a boil; and allow to cook for about two minutes until slightly thickened.

Remove the sauce pan from the heat; carefully stir in vanilla and desiccated coconut.

Pour over pancake or waffles and serve.

Fruit And Nut Oatmeal

Serves 6

Per Serving: Calories: 183 - Fat: 39 - Protein: 69

Ingredients You Will Need

½ cup oat bran, soaked
1 peeled Granny Smith apple, cored and chopped
4 cups coconut water
½ cup raisins or dried cranberries (optional)
1 banana, peeled and sliced
2 cups oatmeal, soaked
1 tsp cinnamon
1 tsp sea salt

Directions

Add to a medium size sauce pan the banana, apple, coconut water, raisins, cinnamon and salt. Place over medium heat and bring to a simmer.

Now, add to the sauce pan the oat bran and oatmeal. Bring to boil for about 3-5 minutes or until the oats are soft. Remove the sauce pan from the fire.

Set aside to cool.

Serve this delicious Fruit and Nut Oatmeal with coconut milk, raw honey and chopped nuts.

Fruit and Coconut Parfait

Serves 5 – 6

Per Serving: Calories: 649 - Fat: 38g - Protein: 12g

Ingredients You Will Need

3 cups fresh mixed berries, (plus 6 additional berries for garnish)
1 ½ cups chopped walnuts
4 ½ cups coconut yogurt
6 bananas, peeled
¾ cup flaxseed
6 tbsps. chia seeds

Directions

Add the chia seeds into the yogurt and mix with a spoon. Pour about ¼ cup of yogurt in the bottom of six glasses.

Now, Layer the ingredients in each glass, adding ¼ cup berries, one tablespoon flaxseed, two tablespoons walnuts, and ½ sliced banana.

Next:

Add another ¼ cup of yogurt and repeat layers. Now, top the parfaits with the remaining ¼ cup yogurt per glass. Garnish with berries.

Serve and enjoy.

Fruit Smoothie

Makes 1 Smoothie

Ingredients You Will Need

Honey (optional)
1 cup fresh strawberries or blueberries
½ ripe banana
1 cup coconut milk

Directions

Place all the ingredients in the refrigerator to chill for two hours before using. You can use frozen fruits also.

Add to a blender the strawberries or blueberries, coconut milk, banana and blend until smooth.

To make the smoothie thick; you can place it into the freezer for 45 minutes to 1 hour before serving. If you like your smoothie sweet, add a small amount of honey to taste.

Yogurt Smoothie

Makes 1 Smoothie

Ingredients You Will Need

1 cup fruit juice
1 cup vanilla yogurt
2 tbsps. melted coconut oil
2 cups fruit

Directions

Place the fruit juice, vanilla yogurt and the two cups of fruit in the refrigerator to chill for about two hours before using.

Frozen fruits can be used also. Add to a blender the fruit, yogurt and juice. Blend until smooth.

Remove the lid from the blender and add the melted coconut oil. Blend for another few seconds.

Coconut Milk Smoothie

Makes 1 Smoothie

Ingredients You Will Need

1 cup orange juice
1 cup coconut milk
1 ripe banana

Directions

Place all the ingredients in the refrigerator to chill for two hours before using.

Add to a blender the orange juice, coconut milk, ripe banana and blend until smooth.

To make the smoothie thick; you can place it into the freezer for 45 minutes to 1 hour before serving.

Hawaiian Sunrise Green Smoothie

Serves 6

Per Serving: Calories: 138 - Fat: 99 - Protein: 29

Ingredients You Will Need

½ cup coconut milk
1 ripe mango, peeled and pitted
1 tbsp. coconut oil
½ ripe avocado, peeled and pitted
1 cup lightly steamed spinach leaves, cooled
½ cup orange juice with pulp
1 banana, peeled

Directions

Add all the ingredients to a blender; cover lid and blend until smooth. Pour into six separate glasses and enjoy.

Coconut Banana Bread

Makes 1 Loaf

Ingredients You Will Need

1 can (5 ½ ounces) crushed pineapple with juice
4 eggs
2 cups sugar
1 cup coconut oil
1 tsp baking soda
1 ripe banana, mashed
4 cups flour
¾ tsp salt
2 teaspoons baking powder
1 cup shredded coconut (unsweetened)

Directions

Set the oven to 350 degrees F. and leave to preheat. In a medium size bowl mix together the sugar and coconut oil. Add to the same bowl the banana, eggs and pineapple with juice. Stir with a spoon.

Next:

Add to the same bowl the coconut, salt, flour, baking soda and baking powder. Mix and combine well.

Now, pour the batter into 2 greased and floured 9" x 5" loaf pans.

Place the baking pan inside the oven and allow to bake for 60 minutes, or until knife or toothpick inserted in the center comes out clean.

Remove from the oven and place it on a large wide dish and cut into 16 ½ -inch slices.

Coconut Recipes

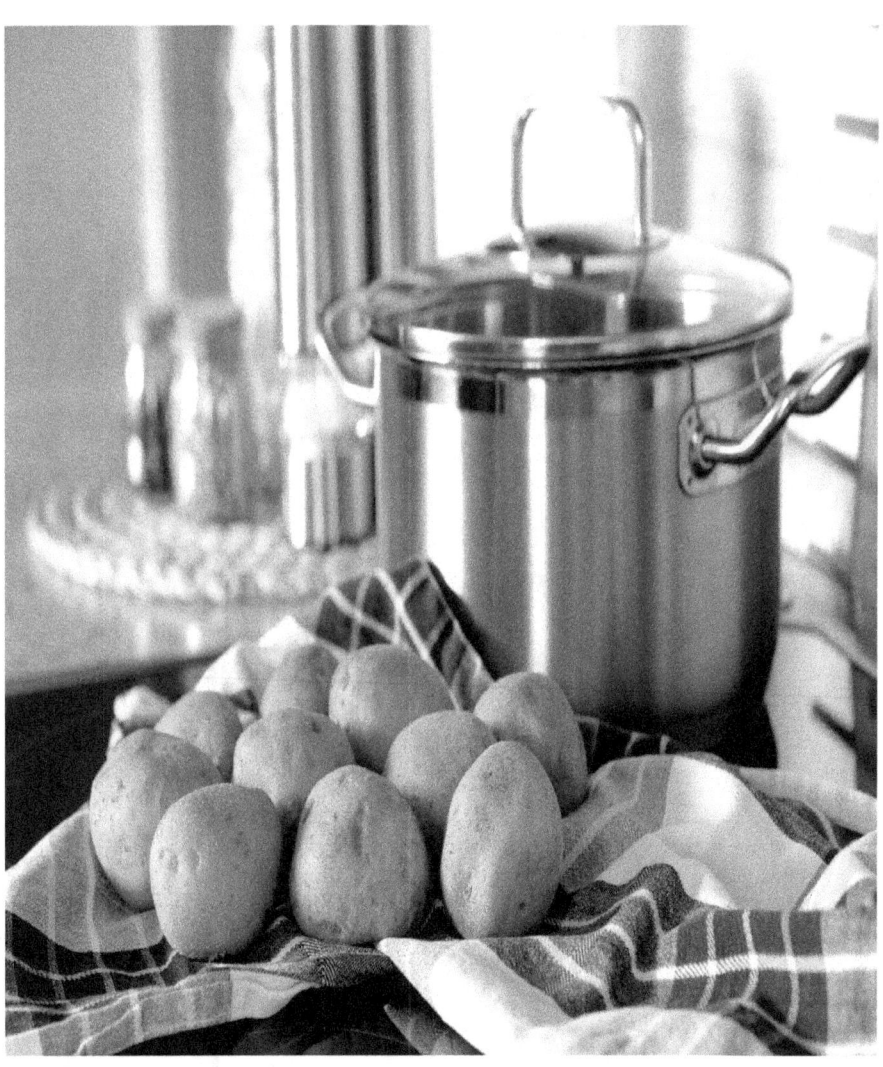

Coconut Cookies

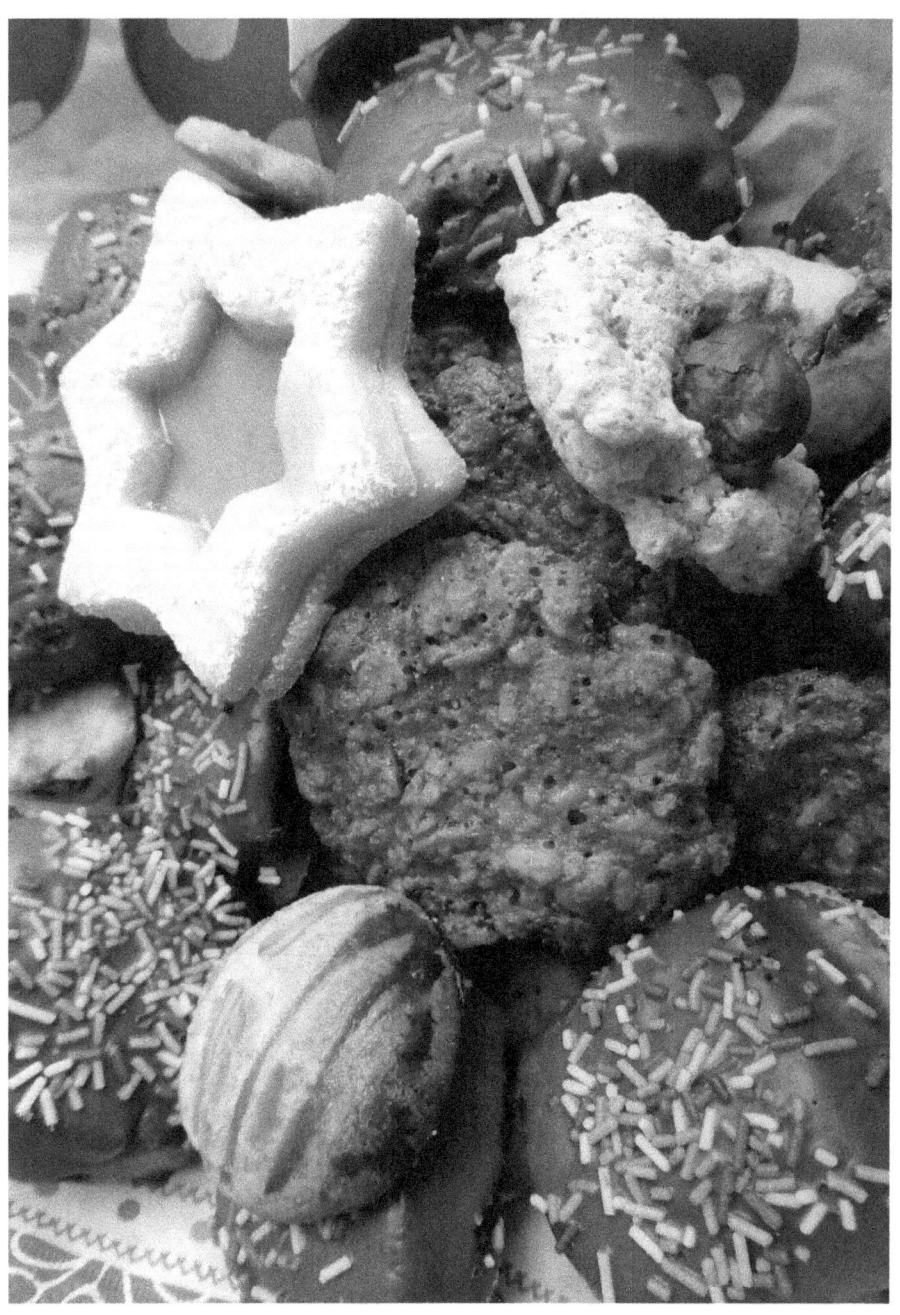

Coconut Oatmeal Cookies

Makes 23 – 25 Cookies

Ingredients You Will Need

1 cup oats
2 large eggs
½ cup coconut oil
½ cup walnuts, finely chopped
½ tsp vanilla extract
1 ½ cups flour
½ tsp baking soda
1 cup brown sugar
½ cup grated coconut
¼ tsp salt
½ tsp cinnamon

Directions

Preheat the oven to 375 degrees F. In the meantime. Mix in a bowl the coconut oil, vanilla, sugar and eggs.

Use a separate bowl to mix together the oats, baking soda, salt, cinnamon, grated coconut and flour. Now, gentle stir in the wet mixture in the bowl, stir well. Now, fold in the walnuts.

Next step.

Set aside the ungreased cookie sheet. Now, roll dough into one and a half inch balls and then place on the cookie sheet. Leave two inches of space between each cookie.

Place the cookies inside the oven and leave to bake for 15 minutes or until golden.

Coconut Cookies

Makes 37 to 41 Cookies

Each Cookie Is Approximately ½ Tablespoon Coconut Oil

Ingredients You Will Need:

3 eggs
1 ½ cups of sugar
3 cups of flour
1 ½ tsp baking powder
1 ½ tsp almond extract
1 tsp salt 1 ¼ cups of coconut oil
1 ½ cups of grated coconut

Direction:

Preheat the oven to 375 degrees F. In the meantime. Mix in a bowl the grated coconut, salt, baking powder and the flour. Set aside. Add to a blender or food processor the eggs, almond extract, coconut oil and sugar. Blend well. Now mix the dry and wet ingredients together in a bowl. Set aside your cookie sheet.

Now roll dough into one and a half inch balls and then place two inches apart on the cookie sheet.

Next step.

Flatten the balls to around half an inch in thickness. Place the cookies in the oven and leave to bake for 12 to 16 minutes, or until golden.

Remove the cookies from the oven and place it on a wire rack to cool.

Main Dish

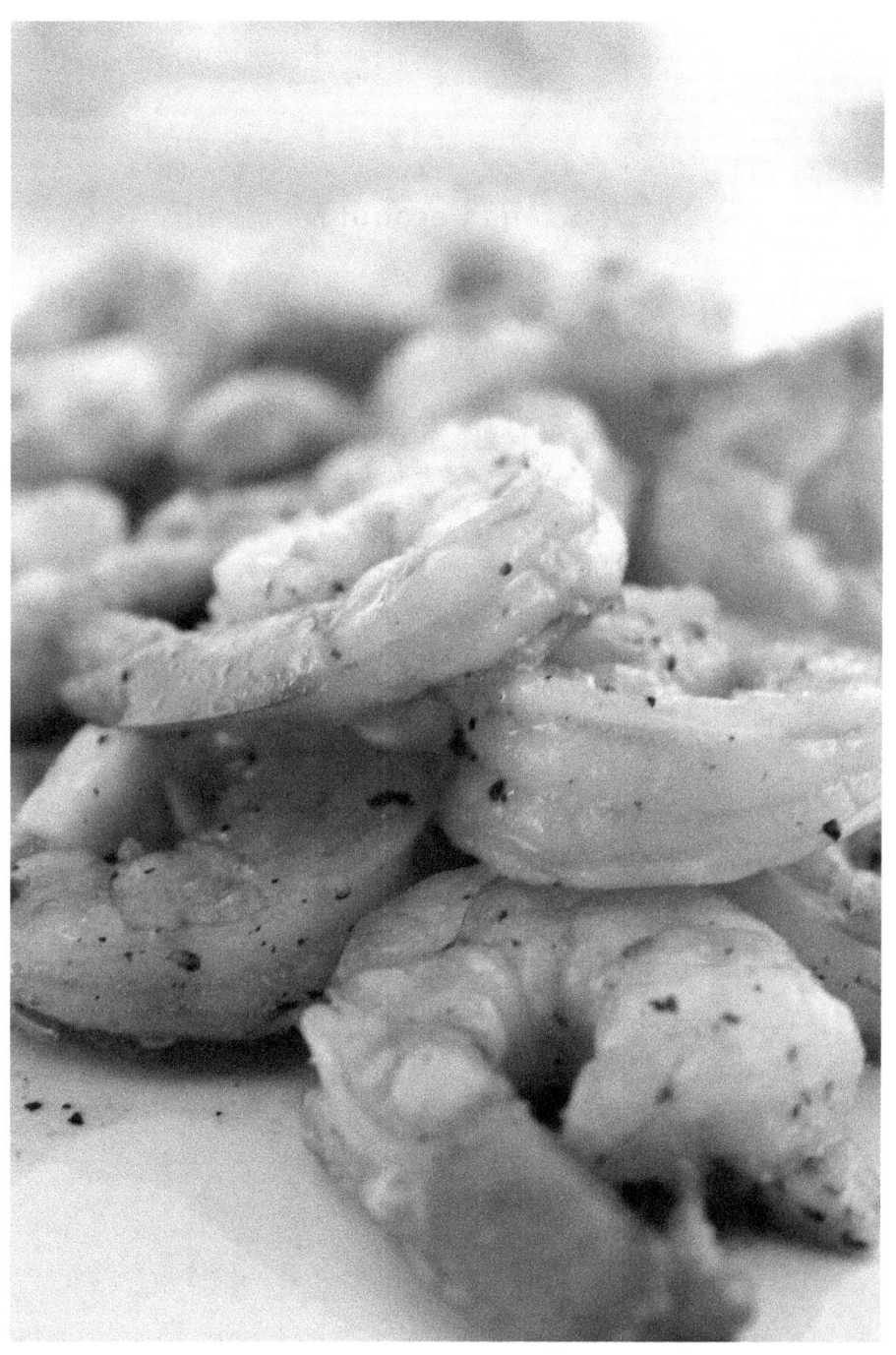

Delicious Coconut Meatballs

Serves 5-6

Ingredients You Will Need

2 large eggs
3 tbsps. Coconut oil
1 large onion (chopped)
1 tsp potato starch flour
Fresh cilantro, (finely chopped) to your taste
2 garlic cloves (chopped or pressed)
½ tsp salt
2 lb. ground beef
1 tsp ground cumin
¼ tsp cayenne
½ oyster sauce
1 tsp coriander
1 cup coconut milk, (divide into 2 portions, you will need the second half for later)
½ cup Portobello mushrooms, (chopped)
1 tbsp. cold water

Directions

Set gas mark to low. Place the skillet on the fire, and pour the coconut oil in. In the meantime. Add to a large bowl the garlic, onions, cumin, eggs, salt, and 4 tbsps.

Coconut milk, coriander, oyster sauce, cayenne and ground beef. Combine and mix well. Now, shape the mixture into one inch balls.

Turn the heat up under the skillet. Place the meatballs inside the skillet and cook 5 – 6 minutes or until golden brown.

Next step.

Carefully remove the meatballs from the skillet. Now add the mushrooms to the skillet. Leave to cook for 2 – 3 minutes. Now, add the remaining coconut milk to the mushrooms and stir.

Next step.

Add to a small bowl the potato starch flour, and water. Now add this to the skillet and bring to a simmer. Leave to cook for another 3 – 4 minutes.

Serve meatballs hot with your favorite rice, top with the cilantro and coconut mushroom sauce.

Slow Cooked Beef Curry

Serves 7-8

Per Serving: Fat: 329 - Calories: 407 - Protein: 239

Ingredients You Will Need

2 tsp curry powder
1 2-pound pot roast
1 large can coconut milk
2 cloves garlic, minced
Salt and pepper
2 tbsps. Fresh ginger, grated
2 large onions, quartered
1 tbsp. ground coriander seed
1 tbsp. coconut oil
1 tbsp. chili pepper flakes

Directions

Place a large skillet over medium to high heat. Pour in coconut oil. Wait until the skillet is very hot. Add the beef to the skillet and brown on each side for about 2-3 minutes. Now, carefully remove the beef from skillet and then transfer it into slow cooker with the onions.

Next:

Add to a medium size bowl the garlic, coconut milk, coriander, chili pepper, ginger, curry, salt, and pepper. Mix well. Now, pour the mixture over the beef.

Leave to slow cook on low heat for 7-8 hours.

Coconut Sauce With Peanut And Chicken Satay

Serves 6-7

Per Serving: Protein: 379 - Calories: 318 - Fat: 159

Ingredients You Will Need

3 tbsps. raw coconut sugar
2 lbs. boneless, skinless chicken breast
2 tbsps. fresh lime juice
2 tbsps. curry paste
1 can coconut milk
1 tsp. fresh ginger, grated
2 cloves garlic, minced
½ tsp. red pepper flakes
3 tbsp. creamy peanut butter

Directions

You will need a food processor or blender.

Add to a food processor the lime juice, coconut sugar, coconut milk, red pepper flakes, peanut butter, ginger, curry paste and garlic. Empty the sauce from the food processor into a large bowl and set aside. Now, cut the chicken into one inch cubes. Now, add the chicken cubes to the sauce you set aside and marinade the chicken with it. Leave it to marinade for at least 45minutes to one hour.

Next:

You will need six wooden skewers for the chicken. Now, thread 6-7 cubes of chicken on each skewer and lay them on a broiler pan.

Cook skewers under the broiler for seven to eight minutes, turning occasionally or until the chicken is properly cooked through and browned.

Lay the skewers on a large plate or platter.

Serve with the peanut coconut dipping sauce and salad on the side.

Chunky Garlic Chicken Bites

Serves 6

Per Serving: Calories: 347 - Fat: 26g - Protein: 20g

Ingredients You Will Need

1 pound chicken breast, Chopped in Chunks
2 tbsps. Coconut milk
½ cup coconut flour
1 egg, beaten lightly
1 cup unsweetened shredded coconut
 ½ cup coconut ghee, melted
¼ tsp garlic powder
¼ tsp black pepper
½ tsp salt

Description

Set oven to 400°F. Leave to preheat. In the meantime, beat the egg and coconut milk together in a large bowl. Get another medium size bowl and mix together the salt, pepper, coconut flour, garlic powder and coconut.

Dip the chicken into egg mixture and then into the coconut mixture.

Now, place the chicken on baking sheet and drizzle with ghee. Put the tray with the chicken into the oven and allow to bake 20 minutes, or until the chicken bites are browned and cooked through properly.

Remove from the oven. Serve with delicious spicy coconut dipping sauce

Coconut Sauce With Sweet And Sour Pork

Serves 5 – 6

Per Serving: Protein: 32g - Calories: 396 - Fat: 20g

Ingredients You Will Need

¾ cup coconut vinegar
2 bay leaves
1 tsp paprika
1 tsp cracked black pepper
 Sea salt, to your taste
2 tbsps. Coconut oil
1 tbsp. raw coconut sugar
1 cucumber, peeled and diced
1 clove garlic, crushed
2 pounds ½ cup creamed coconut lean pork, cut into bite-sized pieces
1 small bunch chives, chopped
2 cups chicken stock
2 firm tomatoes, diced
1 half ripe papaya, peeled, seeded, and roughly chopped

Directions

Add the black pepper, paprika, garlic, bay leaves, vinegar and coconut sugar in a large re-sealable plastic bag.

Mix the ingredients well. Now add the pork to the bag. Leave to marinate for at least 2 hours or more. Place a large skillet over medium to high heat.

Mix the chicken stock as well as the creamed coconut to the skillet. Now, add the pork and leave to simmer for half an hour. Remove pork and coconut sauce from skillet and set aside.

Next:

Mix the tomatoes, cucumber and chives in a small bowl. Set aside. Now, place a skillet on medium fire and add the coconut oil; return pork to the pan.

Cook for another 3-4 minutes, or until browned.

Next:

Add the coconut sauce back to the skillet with the pork. Now, add sea salt to taste along with the papaya.

Cover the pan and leave to cook for another 12-15 minutes.

Serve with cucumber mixture.

Garlic Herb Crackers

Serves 6

Per Serving: Calories: 51 - Fat: 29 - Protein: 39

Ingredients You Will Need

1 tbsp. flaxseeds
¼ tsp garlic powder
½ cup coconut flour
1/8 tsp dried basil
3 tbsps. Water
1 tbsp. sesame seeds
1 tsp virgin coconut oil
2 ½ tsp active dry yeast
1/8 tsp rosemary
¼ tsp salt

Directions

Set oven to 350°F. Leave to preheat. Add to a food processor the flaxseeds, garlic powder, coconut flour, dried basil, sesame seeds, virgin coconut oil, active dry yeast, rosemary, salt.

Note. Don not add the water. Mix well. Now add the water, a little at a time until dough forms. Remove the mixture from food processor. Form into a ball.

Next:

Dust your work surface with a small amount of flour (always clean your surface first). Use a rolling pin to roll out the dough to about ¼ " thick.

Next:

Use a pastry cutter or a sharp knife to cut the dough into one inch squares. Punch four small holes in each square. This will prevent the dough from curling or bubbling on the edges. Set aside your tray.

Next:

Now, arrange squares on the baking tray. Place the tray into the oven and leave to bake for 15 minutes, or until golden brown around the edges.

After 15 minutes; remove from the oven and leave to cool.

Pineapple-Cilantro Dip With Shrimp

Serves 6

Per Serving: Calories: 210 - Fat: 139 - Protein: 69

Ingredients You Will Need

2 large eggs
1 cup bread crumbs
12 large shrimp, peeled and deveined
4 tbsps. Coconut milk
1/3 cup coconut flour
½ coconut, shredded
Coconut oil, as needed
2 cloves garlic
1 jalapeno pepper, seeded
1 cup fresh pineapple, cubed
¼ cup cilantro, chopped
Salt and black pepper, to taste

Directions

Set oven to 400°F. Leave to preheat. In the meantime. Add to a food processor or blender the salt and pepper, bread crumbs and shredded coconut. Blend well.

Place in a large bowl. Set aside. In another medium size bowl, add the coconut flour. Get another small/medium size bowl and whisk the coconut milk and eggs together. Mix well.

Next:

Coat each shrimp in flour. Dip in egg mixture. Dip in coconut mixture. Get a large heavy-bottomed skillet about half inch deep.

Pour coconut oil to cover the bottom of the skillet. Allow the oil to get hot. When the oil is hot, add the shrimp and sauté until golden brown.

Fry on each side for one minute. When the shrimp is cooked through properly, remove and place on a paper towel to drain.

Next:

Now, in a blender or food processor, add the garlic, jalapeno, cilantro, and pineapple. Pulse until coarsely chopped. Serve with shrimp.

Bacon Ginger Mussels

Serves 6

Per Serving: Calories: 164 - Fat: 99 - Protein: 149

Ingredients You Will Need

3 tsps. Fresh ginger, grated
10 – 12 slices thick-cut bacon
3 pounds small mussels
1 tbsp. soy sauce
2 cups coconut water

Directions

Place a heavy-bottomed skillet over medium to high fire. Now, cut the bacon strips in half lengthwise then cut into half inch pieces. Place the bacon in the hot skillet and fry until nearly crisp. Carefully, pour the grease off.

Next:

Turn the heat down to low under the skillet. Now, add to the skillet; ginger, soy sauce and coconut water.

Cover and simmer for about two minutes. After two minutes; turn the heat up to medium high.

Next:

Add the mussels to the skillet and cover. Leave to cook for about 6-10 minutes. Shaking the skillet occasionally, until mussels open.

Remove any mussels that do not open. After 6-10 minutes; transfer the mussels into a bowl and pour coconut bacon broth over the top.

Fried Eggplant

Serves 6

Per Serving: Calories: 309 - Fat: 239 - Protein: 79

Ingredients You Will Need

Coconut oil, (as needed)
2 tbsps. Coconut milk
3 large eggs
3 medium eggplants
½ cup coconut flour
½ tsp. garlic powder
1 tsp. sea salt
½ tsp. black pepper

Directions

Add to a small bowl the coconut milk and eggs. Whisk together until well blended. Get another large bowl and mix the garlic powder, coconut flour, salt and pepper.

Place the eggplant on a flat surface and slice into ¼ " slices. Now, dip the slices into the egg mixture and then into the coconut flour mixture.

Next:

Heat a large skillet on fire. Pour coconut oil to cover the bottom. Wait until the oil is hot enough.

Carefully, place the eggplant in the hot oil and sauté for 3 minutes or until golden brown. Turn and repeat on the other side.

Next:

Transfer to a paper towel and allow it to drain. Serve with coconut dipping Sauce.

Cilantro Crab Dip

Serves 6

Per Serving: Calories: 232 - Fat: 119 - Protein: 179

Ingredients You Will Need

1 pound crab meat
¼ cup cilantro
1 bag plantain chips
1 tbsp. hot sauce
Juice of 2 freshly squeezed limes
1 cup unsweetened coconut milk
½ tsp salt
Freshly ground black pepper, to taste

Directions

Set aside 6 sprigs of cilantro to use as a garnish for later. Chopped the remaining cilantro finely. In a medium size bowl, mix well the hot sauce, coconut milk, lime juice and cilantro. Add to the bowl the salt and pepper.

Next:

Gentle stir in the crab meat. Set aside for about ten to fifteen minutes. Now, Use a spoon to scoop the crab meat into 6 separate serving bowls.

Garnish with the remaining sprigs of cilantro. Serve with plantain chips and enjoy.

Cashew Shrimp Balls

Serves 6

Per Serving: Calories: 412 - Fat: 359 - Protein: 169

Ingredients You Will Need

1 ½ cups cooked shrimp, peeled
¼ cup mango salsa
½ cup cashew pieces (finely chopped)
2 green onions (finely chopped)
2 packages cream cheese
½ cup unsweetened shredded coconut

Directions

Set oven to 350°F. Leave to preheat. On a baking tray, place cashews and coconut. Place inside the oven and leave to bake for three to five minutes or until golden brown. Add to a food processor or blender the salsa, onions, cream cheese and shrimp. Blend well.

Next:

Place cream cheese mixture in the refrigerator for at least one hour. Now, shape into one inch balls; roll in toasted coconut cashew mixture.

You can serve this with Serve with plantain chips.

Roasted Coconut Chicken

Serves 6

Per Serving: Calories: 368 - Fat: 329 - Protein: 199

Ingredients You Will Need

2 tbsps. curry paste
2 tbsps. coconut oil
1 tsp fresh ginger, grated
1 tsp lemongrass, finely chopped
1 (13.5-ounce) can coconut milk
1 large roaster chicken

Directions

Set oven to 350°F. Leave to preheat. Mix and combine the coconut oil, lemon grass, curry paste and ginger with two tbsps.' coconut milk. Using a basting brush; gentle brush the mixture over the chicken.

Next:

Place the chicken in a large roasting pan, and pour remaining coconut milk over the chicken.

Place the chicken inside the oven and leave to roast one and half hours. Baste the chicken occasionally with coconut milk.

After one and a half hours; remove the chicken from the oven and set aside for about seven to eight minutes before carving.

Coconut Rice And Beans With Jerk Chicken

Serves 4

Ingredients You Will Need

Splash of rum.
2 chili pepper, (stemmed and chopped, habanero, Jalapeno)
1 whole lime, juiced
8 cloves garlic, finely minced
3 lbs. chicken pieces, (drumsticks and thighs)
4 tablespoons soy sauce
½ teaspoon ground nutmeg
4 stalks scallions, (fresh, and finely minced)
2 teaspoons ground ginger
4 tablespoons light brown sugar
3 teaspoons salt
4 teaspoons Caribbean allspice
2 tablespoons oil; you can choose from (olive oil, vegetable oil or peanut oil)
2 teaspoons ground nutmeg
2 teaspoons black pepper
1 teaspoon ground cloves

2 teaspoons ground cinnamon

2 thyme, tablespoons dried

1 cup long-grain rice or brown rice

1 shallots, chopped

1 tablespoon oil (butter is optional)

3/4 cup coconut milk

1 cup water

1 clove garlic, chopped

1 can black beans or (15 Oz's black beans, rinsed and drained)

1 teaspoon salt

Directions

Preheat oven to 350°F.

Add to a large bowl the scallions, de-seeded peppers and the garlic. Now, add to the bowl the soy sauce, brown sugar, dried thyme, spices, oil, and a splash of rum (optional) and lime juice. Combine well.

Next:

Add to the same bowl the pieces of chicken and combine. Now, add the chicken to the bowl and rub the mixture all over the chicken.

Next:

Place a cover on the bowl and put inside the refrigerator to marinate for about three hours.

After 3 hours; remove the chicken from the refrigerator and place it on a baking tray. Leave to bake 44-56 minutes.

Next:

In the meantime. Place a saucepan over medium heat. Add a small amount of oil or butter. Now, add the shallot and garlic and stir, cook for about three minutes or until soft.

Add the washed rice to the saucepan and stir. Now, pour in the water and coconut milk. Add the salt and nutmeg.

Cover with lid. Bring to a boil, and then lower the heat to medium-low.

Next:

When the liquid is absorbed and the rice is tender, about eighteen minutes. Slowly stir in the black beans and cook for another 5-6 minutes.

Stewed Jamaican Chicken

Ingredients You Will Need

1 lime (juiced)
1 cabbage
4 tablespoons coconut oil
3 lbs. chicken (cut in chunks)
1 large tomatoes
½ tablespoons black pepper
2 carrots
2 teaspoons sea salt
2 cups water
1 large onion, chopped
2 cloves garlic (crushed)
1 tablespoons browning
1 sweet pepper
1 thyme (fresh sprig)
1/4 green bell pepper, chopped (use red and green)
1 onions (small)
Coconut oil
1 teaspoon arrowroot powder (or cornstarch)
2 carrots (chopped)
Pepper and salt to taste

Directions

Place the chicken in a large bowl and wash with the lime juice. Remove water and pat dry with a paper towel. Mix in a small bowl the black pepper, browning and sea salt.

Rub the mixture over the chicken, and then cover with lid. Place it inside the refrigerator and leave to marinate for at least 1 hour.

Next:

Place a large frying skillet over high heat. Pour oil in. Wait until it's hot. Add the pieces of chicken to the hot skillet and brown on each side. When the chicken is browned on both sides, transfer to another skillet and set aside.

Next:

Now, add the bell peppers and onions to the same frying skillet. Fry until soft. Now, add the browned chicken pieces, carrots, garlic, water and thyme to the skillet. Gentle stir and cover with lid.

Leave to cook on medium heat for 27 - 43 minutes or until the chicken is tender. Stir occasionally.

Next:

Remove the lid from the skillet and add the cornstarch or arrowroot powder to thicken the brown stew gravy. When the rice is cooked; serve it with the chicken. Serve hot with your favorite side dish or salad.

Chicken Salad

Serves 5 - 6

Ingredients You Will Need

¾ cup Coconut Mayonnaise
2 tbsps. Lemon juice
1 cup diced celery
¼ cup minced Spanish onion or Bermuda
3 cups diced cooked chicken
2 tbsps. Pimiento
¼ cup minced bell pepper
1/8 tsp black pepper or paprika
¼ tsp salt

Directions

Add to a large bowl the; coconut mayonnaise, lemon juice, diced celery, minced Spanish onion or Bermuda, 3 cups diced cooked chicken, pimiento, minced bell pepper, black pepper, salt to taste.

Combine and mix all well. Cover with lid, place inside the refrigerator to chill before serving. Garnish with black pepper or paprika before serving.

Coconut Beef Curry

Serves 5 – 6

Per Serving: Calories: 538 - Fat: 289 - Protein: 379

Ingredients You Will Need

2 pounds stewing beef, cut into ¼ " strips
2 onions, sliced
1 tbsp. coconut oil
1 (13.5-ounce) can coconut milk
2 tbsps. Ground cumin
4 medium potatoes, peeled and cubed
2 cloves garlic, minced
1 tsp cinnamon
1 tbsp. curry powder
1 pound baby carrots, peeled
2 tbsps. Tomato paste
Fresh cilantro, chopped
½ cup water
2 tbsps. Paprika
1 tsp sea salt

Directions

Over medium-high heat; place a large saucepan. Add beef strips and coconut oil. Cook for two to three minutes, or until browned. Now, Add curry powder, onions, garlic, cumin, paprika, cinnamon, and; sauté for two minutes.

Next:

Use a large spoon to remove the beef mixture from the saucepan to your 6-quart slow cooker. Add carrots and potatoes to the slow cooker.

Next:

Mix and Combine coconut milk, tomato paste, sea salt and water in a bowl. Now, add mixture to slow cooker.

Cover with lid and leave to cook on low heat for 9-10 hours; until vegetables are tender. Serve hot on plate, sprinkle fresh cilantro on top.

Coconut Beef Stir-Fry

Serves 5 – 6

Per Serving: Calories: 192 - Fat: 129 - Protein: 179

Ingredients You Will Need

¼ cup coconut milk
1 tbsps. ground turmeric
1 tbsp. chili powder
1 pound flank steak
2 tbsps. fresh ginger, minced
3 cloves garlic, minced
½ tsp. dried crushed red pepper
1 onion, halved and sliced
¼ cup fresh cilantro, chopped
 2 tbsps. Coconut oil, melted and divided
1 tsp dark sesame oil

Directions

Cut steak diagonally across grain to cook quicker. Slice thinly into 1/8 inches slices. Rub chili powder and turmeric all over the beef slices. Place the beef in a container with lid and allow to chill for 30 - 40 minutes.

Next:

Place a large skillet over medium-high heat. Add one tablespoon of coconut oil in the skillet. Now, add steak to the hot pan. Stir-fry until browned.

Next:

Remove skillet from heat and sprinkle a little sesame oil over steak. Toss to coat. Now, remove the steak from skillet and set aside.

Next:

Add the remaining one tablespoon of coconut oil into the same skillet. Add onion, ginger and garlic. Stir-fry until onion is translucent.

Next:

Slowly stir in the coconut milk. Cook, stirring frequently, for about 3-4 minutes, or until sauce coats the spoon. Now, stir in red pepper, steak, and cilantro. Cook for an additional 1 minute, or until heated through. Serve over rice and enjoy.

Coconut Beef Stroganoff

Serves 5 – 6

Per Serving: Calories: 535 - Fat: 419 - Protein: 299

Ingredients You Will Need

1 tbsp. Worcestershire sauce
1 pound fresh portobello mushrooms, chopped
1 large onion, chopped
2 pounds beef chuck roast, cut into strips
½ cup fresh parsley, chopped
4 tbsps. Coconut oil, divided
2 tbsps. coconut vinegar
½ cup beef stock
1 tbsp. tapioca starch
3 cloves garlic, minced
1 cup Coconut Sour Cream
Salt and pepper, to taste

Directions

Heat three tablespoons of coconut oil in a medium size saucepan. Add onion and garlic pan. Sauté for two minutes, or until onion begins to brown.

Next:

Grease a 6-quart slow cooker with a little coconut oil. Now, add salt and pepper to your taste, beef strips, garlic, onions and mushrooms to slow cooker.

Next:

Mix in a bowl the Worcestershire sauce, vinegar, tapioca starch and beef stock. Now, pour the mixture in the slow cooker. Cover with lid and cook on low heat for about 5-6 hours.

Next:

About 10 minutes before serving; add the chopped parsley and coconut sour cream to the slow cooker and stir. Serve over pasta and enjoy.

Vegetable Beef Stew

Ingredients You Will Need

2 carrots, chopped
½ onion, chopped
½ cup tomato sauce
1 pound beef, cut into bite-size pieces
Salt and pepper
¼ cup coconut oil
2 medium potatoes, chopped"
1 cup green beans
1 tbsp. diced cilantro
3 cups water

Directions

Place a large saucepan with coconut oil over medium heat. Add the beef to the pan and allow to brown on both sides a little.

Next:

Add to the saucepan the carrots and onion and leave to cook until tender, stirring regularly. Now add green beans, potatoes, tomato sauce, and water.

Next:

Cover with lid and simmer for twenty minutes or until vegetables are tender. Now, add to the pan; salt and pepper to your taste and the cilantro. Cook for an additional one minute.

Baked Salmon with Coconut Crust

Serves 5 – 6

Per Serving: Calories: 394 - Fat: 189 - Protein: 479

Ingredients You Will Need

1 tbsp. coconut oil
1 (3-pound) salmon fillet
½ cup dry bread crumbs
2 tbsps. lemon juice
1 cup grated coconut
Salt and ground black pepper, to taste

Directions

Set the oven to 400 degrees F. and leave to preheat. Cut salmon fillet into 6 equal pieces and place on parchment-lined baking sheet. Use a microwave to melt the coconut oil mix with lemon juice.

Next:

Use a basting brush to coat salmon pieces. In a small bowl, mix coconut, pepper, salt and bread crumbs. Now, dip each piece of salmon in the coconut mixture and place it on baking sheet.

Next:

Sprinkle any remaining coconut topping over salmon pieces. Place the baking sheet inside the oven and bake for about fifteen minutes.

Serve hot and enjoy.

Scallops in Coconut Basil Sauce

Serves 5 – 6

Per Serving: Calories: 457 - Fat: 30g - Protein: 40g

Ingredients You Will Need

1 tbsp. fish sauce
1 tbsps. Fresh ginger, grated
3 pounds sea scallops
Juice from 2 limes
2 cans coconut milk
2 tbsps. Fresh basil, chopped
¼ tsp red pepper flakes

Directions

Add to a large saucepan the lime juice, red pepper flakes, 1 can coconut milk and ginger. Bring to a boil and then lower the heat to medium-low. Now, add to the same saucepan the scallops.

Cover with lid and cook for ten minutes, or until scallops are cooked through. Using a slotted spoon, carefully remove the scallops from the saucepan; place in a flat serving dish. Set aside.

Next:

Add the remaining 1 can coconut milk to a separate saucepan; bring to a boil.

Cook over high heat for fifteen minutes, or until liquid is reduced to about 1 ½ cups. Now, add the fish sauce and basil to the mixture.

Pour over scallops and serve.

Caribbean Curry Shrimp Recipe

Ingredients You Will Need

Season for shrimp:

½ tablespoon black pepper
1 lb. raw shrimp, peeled and de-veined
2 teaspoon curry powder
½ teaspoon salt

Curry sauce ingredients:

1 cup Water
½ red bell pepper, julienned
2 tablespoons coconut milk
½ green bell pepper, julienned
1 tablespoons Ketchup
1 Sprig fresh thyme
3 cloves garlic, minced
2 tablespoons cooking oil
½ teaspoon salt
1 tablespoons curry powder
1 tablespoons cornstarch
½ teaspoon Hot pepper sauce
1 small onion, chopped

Directions

Add to a bowl the peeled shrimp and season with curry powder, salt, and black pepper. Set aside. Julienne red bell peppers, green peppers and onion and mince garlic.

Next:

Place a large frying skillet over high heat. Pour cooking oil in the skillet and wait until it's hot.

Now, add the garlic, peppers and onion to the hot oil. Sauté until onion is transparent. Now, add 1 spring of fresh thyme; stirring occasionally. Lower the fire to medium heat and add coconut milk.

Next:

Add to the skillet curry powder, ketchup, salt and hot pepper sauce; stir. Now, add the shrimp to vegetables and sauté until all the shrimp turn pink.

Next:

In a small bowl, mix with a spoon the cornstarch and water. Add the mixture to the rest of the ingredients. Cover with lid and leave to simmer for one minute, or until shrimp are firm and the sauce has thickened. Add a little pepper and salt to taste.

Serve and enjoy.

Seafood Pasta with Creamy Coconut Sauce

Serve 7 – 8

Per Serving: Calories: 635 - Fat: 209 - Protein: 419

Ingredients You Will Need

2 tbsps. Coconut oil
1 tbsp. anchovy paste
24 ounces dry pasta
1 can coconut milk
1 pound large shrimp, peeled and deveined
2 tbsps. fresh basil, chopped
1 pound mussels, sorted and cleaned
1 pound cod, cubed
2 tsps. Potato starch flour
¼ cup chicken broth
1 large white onion, diced
1 tbsp. thyme
salt and pepper

Directions

Pour coconut oil in a large saucepan over medium heat. Add the onion and anchovy paste; sauté for about four to five minutes, or until onion becomes transparent.

Now, add the coconut milk, thyme, seafood and. Cover with lid and bring to a simmer. Cook on low heat for ten to fifteen minutes, until mussels open and shrimp turn pink.

Next:

In a medium size bowl, whisk together the potato starch flour and chicken broth. Slowly whisk into seafood mixture. Add a little pepper and salt to taste.

Lower the heat. To cook the pasta; follow the directions on the packet. Remove any unopened mussels before serving.

Serve this delicious meal with seafood coconut sauce.

Dessert Recipes

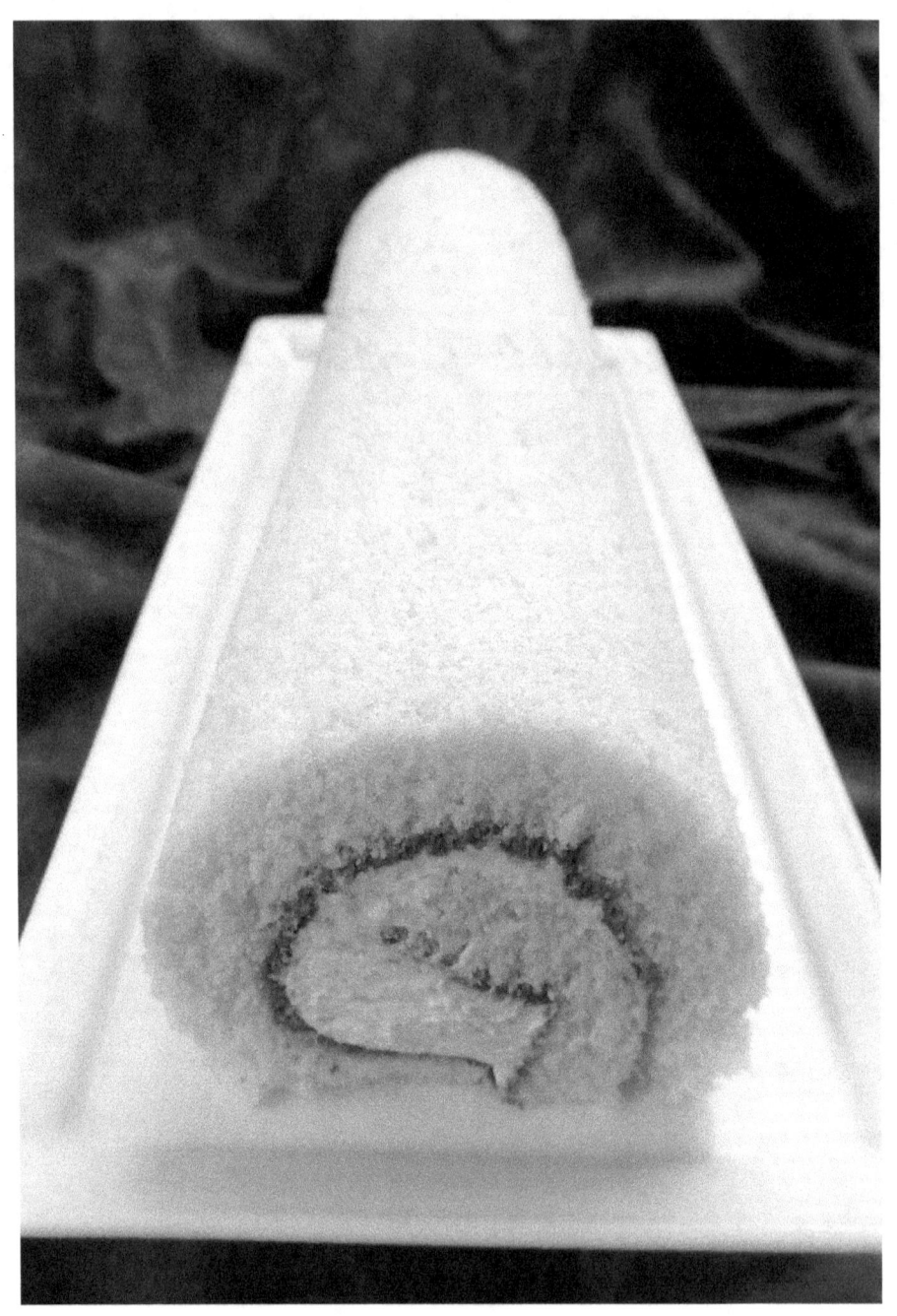

Caribbean Coconut Cake

Ingredients You Will Need

½ teaspoon allspice

1 tablespoon Jamaican rum (this is optional)

1 ½ cups desiccated (unsweetened) or freshly grated coconut

3 cups all-purpose flour

3 teaspoon baking powder

1 teaspoon baking soda

2 cups milk

1 ½ cups brown sugar

½ teaspoon nutmeg

1 teaspoon ground ginger

1 teaspoon vanilla Extract (this is optional)

½ cup raisins (optional)

½ cup butter, melted

2 eggs, well beaten

½ teaspoon Salt

Directions

Set the oven to 350 degrees F. and leave to preheat. Mix all the dry ingredients in a medium to large bowl.

In a separate bowl, beat the milk and eggs together with a fork and then add melted butter. Stir in the rum and vanilla (this is optional).

Next:

Add the wet ingredients to the bowl with the dry ingredients. Mix and combine well until blended. Pour the mixture in a greased 13" x 8" baking pan.

Bake for one hour. Remove from the oven after an hour and place on rack to cool. Cut into squares on a wide dish. Serve and enjoy.

Caribbean Banana Cake

Ingredients You Will Need

⅓ cup walnuts
½ cup walnuts
2 tablespoon milk
1 package Banana Cake Mix
⅓ cup butter flavored shortening
¾ cup brown sugar
1 cup flaked coconut

Directions

Preheat oven to 350°F. In the meantime. Put grease and flour in a 13x9-inch baking pan. In a large bowl, add the cake mix, eggs, oil and water and combine well.

Next:

Use an electric mixer to mix the mixture at medium speed for about two minutes. Now, slowly stir in the ½ cup walnuts, mix it around a bit with a large spoon.

Now, pour the mixture into the greased pan. Place the baking pan inside the hot oven. Allow to bake for 33 to 35 minutes or, you can use a toothpick to insert in the center if it comes out clean then it is cooked.

Next:

Add to a medium size skillet the shortening, coconut, brown sugar, and milk. Mix and combine. Cook the mixture on medium heat, stirring occasionally, until shortening is melted or until golden brown.

Carefully spread over the warm cake. Set the cake on wire rack for 15 minutes to cool.

Serve warm.

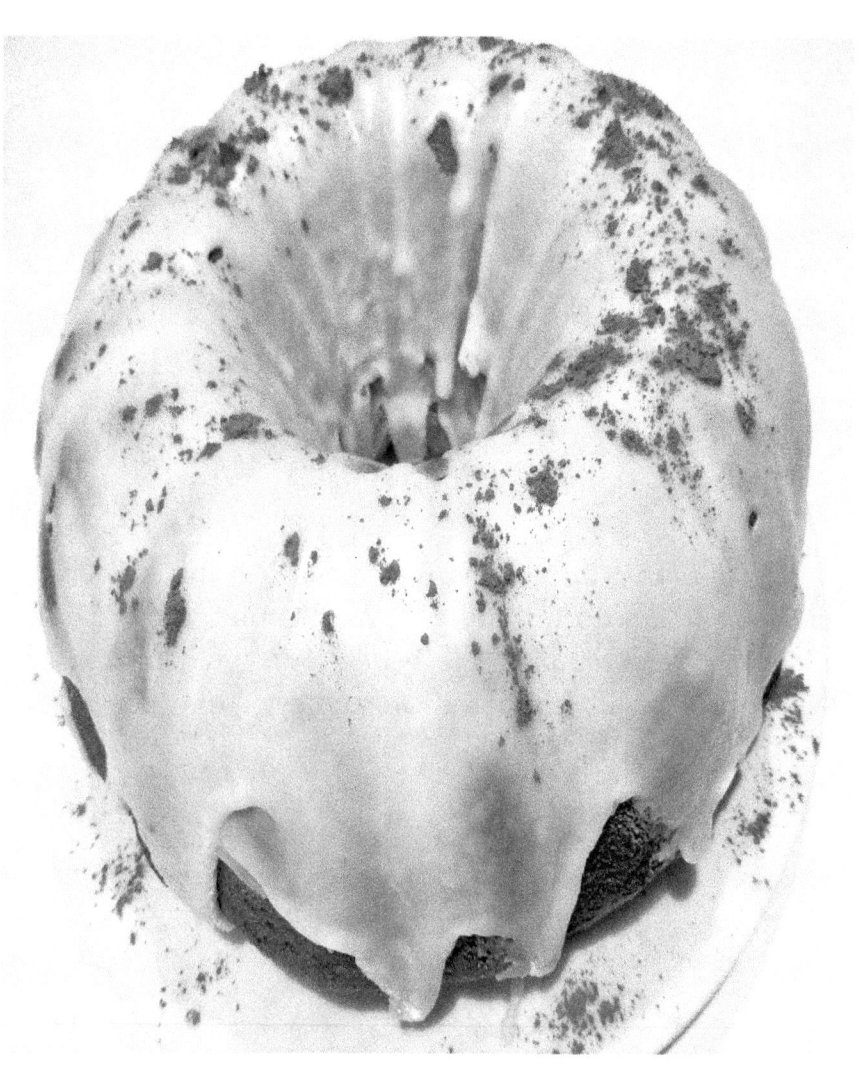

CONCLUSION

So, what are you waiting for? Now that you know what coconut oil can do for you and your family, get yourself a bottle and start reaping the benefits! Your Skin, hair and overall health will thank you! Oh, and even your pets.

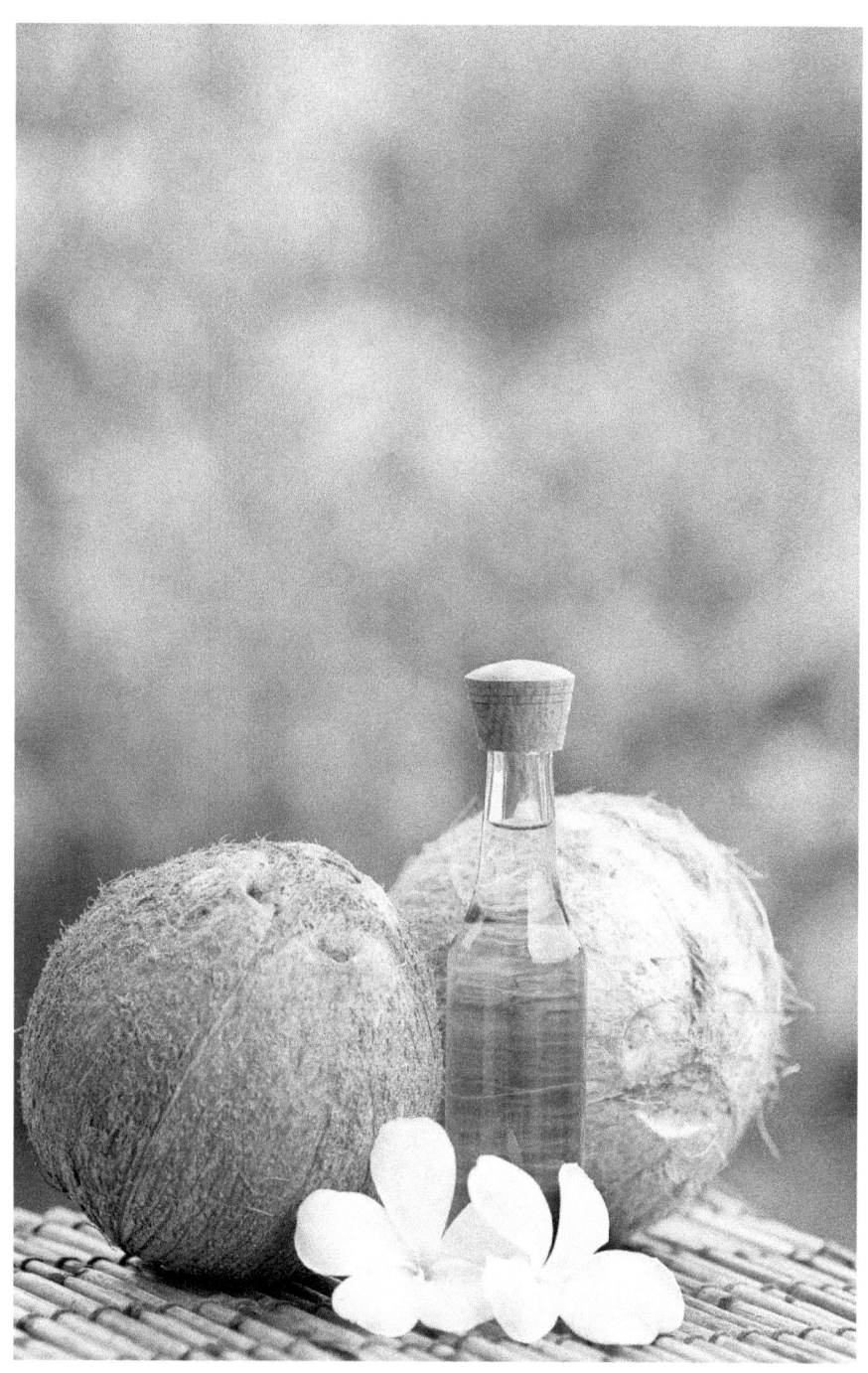

www.ingramcontent.com/pod-product-compliance
Lightning Source LLC
Chambersburg PA
CBHW070916290526
45795CB00001B/330